Health Essentials

Aromatherapy

Christine Wildwood is an experienced aromatherapist. As well as a previous book on aromatherapy, she has written a number of magazine articles on health-related subjects. She also conducts workshops on aromatherapy, deep relaxation and meditation. The author lives in South Wales and runs a very popular aromatherapy and holistic health practice from her home.

The Health Essentials Series

There is a growing number of people who find themselves attracted to holistic or alternative therapies and natural approaches to maintaining optimum health and vitality. The *Health Essentials* series is designed to help the newcomer by presenting high quality introductions to all the main complementary health subjects. Each book presents all the essential information on each therapy, explaining what it is, how it works and what it can do for the reader. Advice is also given, where possible, on how to begin using the therapy at home, together with comprehensive lists of courses and classes available worldwide.

The *Health Essentials* titles are all written by practising experts in their fields. Exceptionally clear and concise, each text is supported by attractive illustrations.

Series Medical Consultant
Dr John Cosh, MD, FRCP

In the same series

Acupuncture by Peter Mole
Alexander Technique by Richard Brennan
Ayurveda by Scott Gerson MD
Chi Kung by James MacRitchie
Chinese Medicine by Tom Williams
Colour Therapy by Pauline Wills
Flower Remedies by Christine Wildwood
Herbal Medicine by Vicki Pitman
Homeopathy by Peter Adams
Iridology by James and Sheelagh Colton
Kinesiology by Ann Holdway
Massage by Stewart Mitchell
Natural Beauty by Sidra Shaukat
Reflexology by Inge Dougans with Suzanne Ellis
Shiatsu by Elaine Liechti
Spiritual Healing by Jack Angelo
Vitamin Guide by Hasnain Walji

Note from the Publisher

Any information given in any book in the *Health Essentials* series is not intended to be taken as a replacement for medical advice. Any person with a condition requiring medical attention should consult a qualified medical practitioner or suitable therapist.

Health Essentials

AROMATHERAPY

Massage with Essential Oils

Christine Wildwood

ELEMENT
Shaftesbury, Dorset • Rockport, Massachusetts
Melbourne, Victoria

© Element Books Limited 1991
Text © Christine Wildwood 1991

First published in Great Britain in 1991 by
Element Books Limited
Shaftesbury, Dorset SP7 8BP

Published in the USA in 1991 by
Element Books, Inc.
PO Box 830, Rockport, MA 01966

Published in Australia in 1992 by
Element Books and distributed
by Penguin Books Australia Ltd
487 Maroondah Highway, Ringwood,
Victoria 3134

Reprinted 1992
Reprinted January and August 1993
Reprinted May and November 1994
Reprinted 1995
Reprinted 1996
Reissued 1997

Cover design by Max Fairbrother
Designed by Nancy Lawrence
Illustrations by David Gifford
Typeset in Goudy by Selectmove Limited
Printed and bound in Great Britain by
Biddles Limited, Guildford and King's Lynn

British Library Cataloguing in Publication
data available

Library of Congress Cataloging in Publication data
Wildwood, Christine
Aromatherapy: massage with essential oils/Christine Wildwood,
(Health essentials series)
Includes bibliographical references and index.
1. Acupressure. I. Title. II. Series.
RM666.A68W55 1991 615'.321–dc20 91–36720

ISBN 1–86204–097–X

Note from the Publisher

Any information given in any book in the *Health Essentials* series is not intended to be taken as a replacement for medical advice. Any person with a condition requiring medical attention should consult a qualified medical practitioner or suitable therapist.

Contents

Acknowledgements

I AM MOST grateful to the following people for responding so speedily and so generously to my requests for further information about essential oils. First, Nick Webley of *Kittywake Oils* (friend and associate), Bernie Hephrun of *Butterbur and Sage*, and Dr Steve Van Toller of Warwick University.

Many thanks also to Robert Tisserand for allowing me to use an abridged version of John's Story from the *International Journal of Aromatherapy*, and to Ellen Asjes for her lovely letter of support. I must also thank my family for the domestic help which enabled me to find time to write this book. Finally, my thanks extend to Karin Cutter and to John – who holds the torch for the future of holistic aromatherapy.

Introduction

ALTHOUGH THE WORD 'aromatherapy' is modern, the roots of this beautiful therapy lie buried in the depths of antiquity. This little book sets out to prove that the ancient principles on which aromatherapy is based are no less valid today. It is also intended as a guide for those wishing to employ aromatic plant essences for pleasure and to promote health and vitality in themselves and their loved ones.

To derive the greatest benefit from the massage section, ideally the reader will have a friend or partner with whom to exchange aromatherapy massage. However, as we shall discover, aromatic essences can be used in many other ways to engender a sense of well-being and to impart an aesthetic element to life.

Although the art of aromatherapy massage could not possibly be explained fully in a condensed book such as this, the basic massage sequence outlined in Chapter 6 will give readers a grounding from which they may begin to develop their own intuitive style. For those wishing to go further, listed in the appendix are some very good training establishments and other useful addresses. There is also a suggested reading list of books on aromatherapy and other relevant subjects.

Aromatherapy, in common with all *holistic* therapies, seeks to strengthen the body's own innate self-healing ability. Even though some people are born healthier than others, most of us can become healthier and prevent the development of serious disorders such as diabetes and heart disease. The key to good health and a sense of well-being lies in the realisation that we need not become helpless victims of stress, or *dis*tress, which accounts for a great deal of illness. To a large extent, of course, our health is dependent on the quality of food we eat, the water we drink and the air we breathe. Perhaps even more importantly, we need to nurture the spiritual aspect of 'self', for we are more than a body and a mind. The spiritual aspect is hard to define, but is tied up with our relationship with ourselves, with other people and with our sense of purpose and meaning – and indeed, with the health of our planet. Therefore, the holistic therapist seeks to address the interrelated aspects of our being as a whole: the body-mind-spirit. Whatever affects one aspect – the body, the mind or the spirit – affects the WHOLE.

My own approach to the art of aromatherapy could be described as holistic/intuitive. This may not be the style adopted by all aromatherapists, but this is the direction I have found suits my own temperament. Most intuitive therapists are aware of the subtle energy field or *aura* surrounding and interpenetrating the physical body. The aura, if healthy, is rather like a protective filter, allowing only that which is beneficial to affect us. However, the field can become weakened by the stresses of life, allowing inharmonious influences that give rise to illness. For this reason, included in Chapter 7 (which explains the holistic concept) are a few spiritual healing techniques which the reader may choose to accept or disregard according to his or her own perspective. For the down-to-earth reader, there is also a great deal of common sense to found in these pages.

IMPORTANT: Information and suggestions in this book are meant as a guide. The reader is advised and encouraged to seek the aid of a qualified therapist or doctor if under medication or suffering from long-term health problems.

Christine Wildwood,
3 November 1990

1

What is Aromatherapy?

Aromatherapy is more than just another alternative therapy. Certainly it is much more than an upmarket beauty treatment, as some would have us believe. Indeed, aromatherapy is an art, an aesthetic healing art which uses essential oils extracted from various parts of aromatic plants and trees to promote health of body and serenity of mind.

Aromatherapy is the only healing art which could be described as creative in an artistic sense. This is because much of the skill of an aromatherapist lies in his or her ability to concoct wonderful aromas by mixing and blending vegetable oils and fragrant essences.

Unlike more clinical therapies such as homeopathy or acupuncture, aromatherapy's healing potential stems from its ability to promote relaxation and, at the same time, to engender a sense of joy or tranquillity in the recipient. Indeed, the more wonderful the experience, the more healing its effect. Perhaps for this reason above any other, aromatherapy has sometimes been dismissed out of hand by a few dyed-in-the-wool traditionalists because they believe a certain amount of discomfort must be felt if it's to do us any good!

Despite one doctors comment 'I know of no specific evidence to show that aromatherapy is of any real clinical value'[1] aromatherapy can indeed be practised on a clinical or down-to-earth scientific level. Dr Kurt Schnaubelt's article Oils for Viral Diseases[2] for instance, gives evidence of the scientific basis of clinical aromatherapy, and already in Germany essential oils are increasingly used to treat viral infections, notably Melissa oil for cold sores. Much more remarkable, essential oils such as tea tree, garlic and thyme have helped a man conquer AIDS! (see page 29).

Before we go any further, it is important to point out here that it would be far too ambitious (and potentially risky) for the lay person and, indeed, the average aromatherapist, to attempt treating serious disorders with essential oils. Aromatherapy, as it is more usually practised, is about *prevention* of major illness and the symptomatic treatment of minor ailments. The emphasis is on aromatherapy massage which is one of the finest techniques available for soothing the detrimental effects of stress. Stress, in its many guises, accounts for the vast majority of ills in this world of speed, 'high-tech' and emotional unrest.

Even though aromatherapy massage is the mainstay of the art, essential oils are used in a variety of other ways for healing and aesthetic purposes – in baths, steam inhalations and as mood enhancing perfumes for example. But in order to fully answer the question 'what is aromatherapy?', we need to take a closer look at these amazing aromatic oils.

ABOUT ESSENTIAL OILS

Essential oils, or essences as they are often called, are the odoriferous, volatile (they readily evaporate) liquid components of aromatic plants. They accumulate in specialised cells or in specific parts of the plant. They may be found in the petals (rose), the leaves (eucalyptus), the wood (sandalwood), the fruit (lemon), the seeds (caraway), roots (sassafras), rhizomes (ginger), resin (pine), gums (frankincense), and sometimes in more than one part of the plant. Lavender, for instance, yields an essential oil from the flowers and leaves. The orange tree is particularly interesting for it produces three different-smelling essences with differing therapeutic properties: neroli (blossom), petit-grain (leaves) and orange (rind).

A plant produces essential oils for its own survival: to influence growth and production; to attract pollinating insects; to repel predators; and to protect itself from disease.

The quality of an essential oil depends on a number of different interacting factors: soil conditions, climate, altitude and the time of harvesting – which is vital. The concentration of essential oil in plants is highest during warm weather and this is the best collecting time. Jasmine, being a night-scented flower, must be picked at dusk.

2

Generally, the harvesting of essential oil plants should be completed within a matter of days; any delay, and the essential oils will be lost. Also, like wine, the quality and 'bouquet' of an essential oil will vary from year to year.

The more oil glands or ducts present in the plant, the cheaper the oil and vice versa. For instance, 100 kilos of lavender yields almost 3 litres of essential oil, whereas 100 kilos of rose petals can yield only half a litre of oil. Although they can be expensive, essential oils are highly concentrated substances; in practice, a little goes a long way.

Although essences are technically classified as oils, they are in fact very different from ordinary 'fixed oils' such as corn or sunflower. Because they are highly volatile they do not leave a permanent mark on paper, and unlike fatty vegetable oils, essences have the consistency of water or alcohol and are not greasy. They are soluble in alcohol, wax (melted beeswax or jojoba for example) and in vegetable oils; because they are *partially* soluble in water, they can be used undiluted in the bath (six drops is usually sufficient) without leaving behind a greasy residue.

HOW THEY ARE EXTRACTED

To many people, this knowledge will be of passing interest. To the environmentally concerned, however, the origin and extraction method for capturing an essence may be of vital importance. Unfortunately, there are many essential oils sold in the aromatherapy market which are not as pure or as natural as generally believed. Some may contain adulterants to enhance the aroma or to extend it so that it goes further; others may contain pesticide residues or traces of chemical solvent from the extraction process. It is possible to obtain aromatherapy grade oils but, before we discuss that, let us take a look at the main extraction methods in operation today.

The most classic method is direct distillation, which is a sophisticated version of the ancient Egyptian clay-pot method. Plant material is placed in the still and is in direct contact with the water. This is heated and steam carries the essential oils into a condenser and then a separator. A far more efficient method, which prevents burning of the distillate, is steam distillation. This is similar to the former method except that plant material does not come into contact with the water; only the steam is passed over it.

A more recent innovation is vacuum distillation. By reducing air pressure inside the sealed distillation apparatus, a vacuum is created. Distillation is thus achieved at much lower temperatures which preserves the delicate flower fragrances more successfully.

The least complicated of the methods is called expression. The essential oil in citrus fruit is found in the outer rind, so simple pressure is used for extracting the oils. Although it was once carried out by hand, machines using centrifugal force are now used instead.

An almost obsolete method of extraction is enfleurage. Animal fat (sometimes olive oil) is used to absorb the essential oils which are then separated from the fat by alcohol. Essences readily dissolve in alcohol, but fat does not. The alcohol is later evaporated off, leaving the essential oil behind. This method is used to capture the fragrances of flowers such as jasmine, tuberose and neroli (orange blossom) whose exquisite fragrances would be spoiled by the intense heat of distillation. The resulting liquid is known as an 'enfleurage absolute' rather than an essential oil. Unfortunately, the high cost of this labour-intensive and time-consuming method has led to the wide use of volatile solvents such as petroleum ether, hexane and benzene as a means for capturing essences of certain flowers – yet the enfleurage process gives a higher yield. Incidentally, it is still possible to obtain enfleurage absolutes of tuberose and jasmine from several French distillers (contact Kittywake Oils, address on page 131). However, the use of pig fat in the enfleurage process will be off-putting to the vegetarian who may have to forego the pleasures of jasmine and tuberose or track down a supplier of the even more elusive vegetable oil absolutes.

Volatile solvent extraction is employed a great deal in the perfume industry because it produces superb fragrances which are truer to the aroma found in the living plant. But should potentially carcinogenic substances such as benzene play any part in the healing art of aromatherapy? Is it not better to use a product with a slightly less than exquisite perfume for the sake of the planet as well as our health?

Quite apart from concern over the traces of solvent often left behind in absolutes, we cannot ignore the environmental effects of solvents being discharged into the atmosphere and possibly being absorbed by distillery workers.

A relatively new but, at present, costly process for capturing precious fragrances is carbon dioxide extraction. This is of great interest from the aromatherapy viewpoint because there is no risk of solvent residues in the resulting extraction. However, whether it is an entirely environmentally friendly process remains to be seen.

WHAT ABOUT ORGANICALLY PRODUCED OILS?

Until very recently the essential oil trade was almost exclusively confined to the perfume and flavours industries – where synthetic or nature identical substances were included without a second thought. However, with the blossoming of interest in aromatherapy, coinciding with green awareness, there is a great demand for pure, unadulterated essential oils – organically produced if possible.

Indeed, it is possible to obtain organic oils from a few suppliers (see page 131), but these essences are considerably more expensive than those from plants grown with chemical fertilizers and sprayed with non-organic pesticides. Moreover, the choice of organic oils is, at present, limited mainly to herbal essences such as lavender, chamomile, thyme and marjoram. However, changes are afoot: organisations such as EOTA (the Essential Oil Trade Association UK) are taking steps to establish reliable sources of pure, unadulterated essential oils for aromatherapy. These oils would have verification of purity from organisations such as the Soil Association in the UK and from others such as IFOAM (International Federation of Organic Agricultural Movements) which exists in Europe and the USA. It is hoped that aromatherapy will benefit from this in two ways: that the purity of an oil can be guaranteed and that there will be a greater choice of organic oils more widely available.

BUYING ESSENTIAL OILS

It is crucial that only pure, unadulterated essential oils are used in therapy. Most aromatherapists obtain their oils from reputable mail order suppliers (see page 131), not from shops concerned with beauty and perfumery. The advantages offered by mail order suppliers over retail outlets include a wider range of oils and lower prices on larger quantities. For the newcomer, however, it may be best to buy essential oils from a health food shop or from a well-respected herbal supplier. This will give you the opportunity of smelling the oils first, and buying only those you like.

Storage is important (see page 47). Essential oils should be sold in well-stoppered, dark-glass bottles and stored away from light, heat and damp. Avoid essential oils sold in bottles with a rubber-tipped dropper. In my experience, certain essential oils, cedarwood in particular, can cause rubber to perish into a sticky mess. Despite this rather alarming fact, essential oils are harmless to skin if used correctly as advocated in this book.

A WORD ABOUT TREE OILS

Due to world-wide excitement about the amazing medicinal properties of tea-tree essence (*Malaleuca alternifolia*), the Brazilian government is seriously considering a massive planting programme of the species, which is native to Australia, in the wastes that were once rainforests.

However, there may be cause for concern over the capturing of rosewood essence (sometimes called Bois de Rose). At present, the principal supplies are from trees grown in Brazil. The essence is distilled from wood used in the Brazilian lumber industry (most of the wood going to US furniture-makers). Tragically, these trees are being torn down from the rapidly diminishing rainforests – and are not being replanted. Until the Brazilian government begins a replanting programme of this species (and indeed, of *all* trees), I for one feel obliged to avoid this oil – including supplies of rosewood from other areas of South America and also Africa.

It is not all gloomy news for trees: the situation regarding Indian sandalwood oil (Mysore) is much healthier. The Indian government has ordered that for every tree felled, two more must be planted in its place – and this is actually happening.

THE PROPERTIES OF ESSENTIAL OILS

All essences are antiseptic; some are endowed with anti-viral or anti-inflammatory properties as well. It is generally believed that garlic and tea-tree essences are the most powerful anti-viral oils. For obvious reasons, garlic essence is not usually employed in aromatherapy massage (though it has been known!) but instead, is taken as a medicine in the form of garlic capsules. Unlike chemical antiseptics, essential oils are harmless to tissue, yet they are powerful aggressors towards germs. Dr Jean Valnet (one of the French pioneers of aromatherapy) used essential oils to treat the horrific war wounds of soldiers during the Second World War. Not only did the fragrances of the essences cover up the putrid smells of gangrenous wounds, they also suppressed them by retarding putrefaction.

Essential oils promote natural healing by stimulating and reinforcing the body's own mechanisms. Essences of chamomile and thyme, for instance, are credited with the ability to stimulate the production of white blood cells which help in our fight against disease. Lavender, in particular, has the remarkable ability to stimulate the regeneration of skin cells – wonderful in the healing of burns, scar-tissue, wounds, ulcers and so forth.

Essential oils also act on the central nervous system – some will relax (chamomile, lavender), others will stimulate (rosemary, basil). A few have the ability to normalise. Garlic, for instance, can raise low blood pressure and lower high blood pressure. Likewise, bergamot and geranium can either sedate or stimulate according to the needs of the individual – a phenomenon totally alien to a synthetic or chemical drug.

The chemistry of essential oils is complex. They may consist of hundreds of components such as terpenes, alcohols, aldehydes, esters and, no doubt, many other as yet undiscovered components. This explains why a single essential oil can help a wide variety of disorders. As essential oils occur in nature (rather than in the laboratory), side-effects are virtually non-existent.

A chemical or synthetic drug may contain a single, therefore an unbalanced, but very powerful active principle. These drugs lack the synergistic (working in harmony) action of an essential oil, homoeopathic remedy or herbal medicine. As a result, they act in the manner of the proverbial sledge-hammer to crack a nut. Adverse side-effects are the inevitable outcome of such an onslaught.

Of course not all substances occurring in nature are benign. We need only think of laurel leaves (from which cyanide is derived) and the foxglove, which can be lethal unless cautiously administered.

However these two plants taken in homoeopathic form cause no problems in toxicity whatsoever.

As a matter of interest, Dr Jean Valnet and other doctors in the field of clinical aromatherapy have discovered that blends of certain essential oils are not only more powerful than when used singly, but that the mysterious factor of synergy is at work – the whole becoming greater than the sum of its equal parts. This is particularly noticeable with the anti-bacterial action of essences. A blend of clove, thyme, lavender and peppermint, for example, is far more powerful than the chemist might expect of the blend (taking into account the combined chemical constituents of the oils). Curiously, rather like a discordant musical note, by mixing more than five essences, the effect is counter-productive. The anti-bacterial action is weakened.

Aromatherapy, in common with other natural therapies, aims to strengthen the immune system. Allopathic (orthodox) medicine tends to weaken the body's defences by suppressing conditions without removing the cause. At the same time, chemical drugs cause side-effects which the body then has to deal with as well as the disease. This can lead to *iatrogenic* disease (drug induced), a problem which may be far more wide-spread than is generally realised.

However, we need to adopt a balanced viewpoint and accept that the use of drugs cannot be totally ruled out; everything has its place in the *holistic* scheme of things. If, for example, a person fails to respond to natural treatment and is in a great deal of discomfort, or in life or death situations (road accidents, congenital organ dysfunction, and so forth) drug intervention may be vital.

AROMATHERAPY IN PRACTICE

The most fascinating aspect of aromatherapy is the influence of aroma on the mind and emotions – and herein lies the mysterious potency of the art. Indeed, this influence of aroma on the psyche has led some aromatherapists to practise what is now called 'psycho-aromatherapy', whereby oils are used solely as mood altering substances. Other aromatherapists adopt an intuitive approach to the art, preferring not to choose appropriate oils for a client, but to allow the person to be guided solely by their aroma preference. More often than not, oils chosen this way turn out to be the very ones needed at the time, and as the person's physical

8

and emotional state alters, so might their aroma preference. Mind and body are interrelated: whatever affects one will also affect the the other.

NATURAL VERSUS SYNTHETIC

Although chemists have tried to duplicate essential oils in the laboratory, they are not the same. A synthetic chemical is, in theory, identical to that found in nature; in practice, as every chemist knows, it is impossible to make a 100 per cent pure chemical. Any synthetic chemical will carry with it a small percentage of undesirable substances which are not found in the essential oil. Moreover, it lacks the vital enzymes and probably a multitude of other substances in plants as yet undiscovered. But above all, a synthetic chemical lacks the life-force found only in nature. No synthetic chemical or compound can reproduce the vibration or pattern of the 'stuff of life'.

Turning from aromatherapy for a moment, one good example of the natural clearly winning over the synthetic is to be found in the case of insulin. At the time of writing, synthetic insulin – which to the scientist is chemically identical to that secreted in the pancreas – cannot be administered to diabetic people because it simply does not work; yet pig's insulin injected into the human body does!

In the western world the education system is geared to the over-development of left-brain activity (logic) at the expense of the more mystical right-side. This means we tend to mistrust intuition, philosophy and abstract concepts (what the Chinese call the 'yin' or feminine principle) in favour of technology, mathematics and all that is measurable (or, as the Chinese call it, the yang or masculine principle). This results in a materialistic society that worships consumer goods, and where academics rule rather than artists and philosophers. The ideal situation would be a marriage between the two seemingly opposing principles, where alternative and orthodox practitioners reign harmoniously side by side. Just as day cannot exist without night or the Sun without the Moon, logic is dehumanised without the balance of intuition and feeling.

Our intuition tells us that the use of synthetic oils is antithetical to the philosophy of aromatherapy – even though some synthetic oils contain 'active principles' derived from plants. In the words of the great philosopher Rudolph Steiner (1861–1925), 'Matter is the most spiritual in the perfume of the plant.' And it is this spiritual thread which runs through, and on one level, unites all natural healing philosophies. In acupuncture it is called *chi*, in Ayurvedic medicine (from India) it is *prana*, in Reichian Psychotherapy it is *orgone*. In many other schools of thought is is simply 'energy' or 'spirit'.

To the materialist, all this talk of 'life-force', 'spirit' and 'energy' may seem like mumbo-jumbo, totally removed from reality, but reality is more than three-dimensional. Like a beautiful fragrance, spiritual reality needs to be experienced in order to be appreciated; it is impossible to put into words. Spiritual reality is an intuitive, rather than an intellectual knowing. It cannot be measured by scientific instruments – and here we must leave it!

2

A Brief History

THE TRUE ORIGINS of aromatherapy have evaporated into the mists of time. Since the dawning of history, people have been fascinated, intoxicated and mystified by the powers of aromatic plants. Although the word aromatherapy was coined in the 1920s by the French chemist René Gattefossé, first we shall aim the historical telescope much further back in time to The Beginning.

Our early ancestors lived in a world fraught with danger; yet they were far more advanced in the art of survival than many of us in the modern world could ever envisage. Contrary to popular belief, it was not merely by chance, or even more crudely, by a game of Russian Roulette, that our ancestors singled out the edible and medicinal plants from those that were poisonous. They were almost certainly endowed with highly developed sensory and intuitive powers seen only in the few remaining native tribes alive today.

You may have heard reports of American Indian hunters, for example, who are able to follow prey for long distances by using their senses, particularly the sense of smell. They can even distinguish the scent of other human beings by sniffing the ground where they may have walked. Likewise, our early ancestors most probably sifted out the useful plants by scent, sight and intuition. In other words, by instinct.

To dispel another myth: we have not entirely evolved from this animal ability to use our senses for survival. It is merely a case of conditioning and adaptability. A super-efficient sense of smell is no longer vital to our existence. However, when circumstances arise to make it so, then a different pattern emerges. In his book *Body Power*,

11

Dr Vernon Coleman cites the case of an American prisoner who had developed considerable hunting skills. He was able to identify warders by their scent, breathing patterns and the sound of creaking joints as they walked. He could even smell a packet of cigarettes hidden in a coat pocket several metres away!

As well as discovering edible and medicinal plants, our early ancestors discovered something even more interesting: that certain aromatic plants, when burnt on the fire, gave rise to altered states of consciousness. It was found that some aromas made people feel drowsy, others made them feel uplifted or even euphoric. The most precious of all gave rise to mystical or psychic experiences. These were highly prized and burnt only by the priests or priestesses during magical rites, worship of the gods or for healing purposes. Since healing and religion were interrelated, the smoking of sick people (to exorcise evil spirits) became one of the earliest forms of medicine. Juniper, for instance, was a special plant associated with purification, particularly around the symbolic time of the death and rebirth of the Sun at the Winter Solstice. Even after the disappearance of the Druidical priesthood, native Celtic country folk continued to use juniper for ritual fumigations in order to wipe out disease.

Incidentally, fumigation with aromatic substances to prevent the spread of infectious disease is still used in certain parts of the world, and up until relatively recently, French hospitals burnt juniper, thyme and rosemary in the wards as a disinfectant.

On another level, frankincense, the most commonly used incense in churches, has the ability to deepen the breathing. Deep breathing calms the mind and relaxes the body, thus creating a state inducive to prayer and meditation.

The Ancient Egyptians are generally regarded as the true founders of aromatherapy. Aromatics were used in magic and healing (which included different forms of massage) and for cosmetics and embalmment. Indeed, the well-preserved mummies of animals, pharaohs and queens on display in many museums bear witness to the skills of the ancient Egyptian embalmers and to the remarkable preservative powers of plant essences.

As a matter of interest, I once met a forensic scientist fortunate enough to have been present during a research experiment in which a mummy was unwrapped. He and his colleagues were intrigued by the aromas of cedarwood and myrrh which were still perceptible on the inner bandages after nearly 3,000 years!

The botanical gardens of Egypt were a wonder to behold. Many rare and beautiful plants were collected from distant lands such as India and even China. They were made into medicines, perfumes and unguents by the Egyptian priests and priestesses who became so renowned for their skills that sages and physicians from all over the ancient world came to Egypt to study medicine and the Mysteries.

Most archaeologists believe the Egyptians did not use essential oils as such (captured by distillation) but that plants and gums were made into oils and unguents by infusing them. This means placing the plant material in a base of oil or fat and leaving the mixture in the sun for a few days. After this time, the base becomes permeated with the aroma.

However, according to Dr Jean Valnet,[3] the Egyptians used a primitive form of distillation to extract the essential oils from plants. Water was poured into large clay pots over the plant material (usually cedarwood) and the pot openings were covered in woollen fibres. The pots were heated and the essential oils rose in the steam and became lodged within the wool. This was later squeezed to obtain the essential oil. Oil of cedarwood was highly prized for its use in embalmment, medicine and perfumery. It was also the most expensive and sought-after perfume in the whole of the ancient world.

Incidentally, similar distillation pots have been found at Tepe Gawra, near ancient Nineveh. They are thought to date back to 3,500 BC, which suggests that the technological achievements of the Mesopotamians have been grossly underrated. The discovery of distillation is usually accredited to the Arabs of the eleventh century AD.

Another Egyptian method for extracting essential oils from flowers was by squeezing. A bas-relief, now in the Louvre in Paris, depicts women gathering lilies into a large cloth bag, while two men hold sticks attached to the sides of the bag. These sticks would be twisted round until the bag was tightly pressed and the essential oil oozed out of the petals.

Piles of aromatic substances such as frankincense, myrrh, juniper and cypress were burnt in the city squares during important festivals to purify the air and to allow the common people to enjoy breathing in the aromatic smoke. A favourite incense burnt in the temples and at state ceremonies was Kyphi, a luxurious and heady brew consisting of up to sixteen ingredients which included saffron, cassia, spikenard, cinnamon and juniper. The whole compound was bound together with honey and raisins. Dioscorides said it was a perfume welcome to the gods. Kyphi was always burnt after sunset for its effects were soporific and intoxicating.

In ancient China, herbal medicine was used in conjunction with acupuncture and massage to treat a myriad of ailments. However, the Chinese were also involved with the quest for immortality through the practice of alchemy.

The alchemist would burn incense and douse himself in specially prepared perfumes before carrying out his experiments. He believed that the perfume of plants held magical forces and plant spirits whose power would help him concoct the elixir of life.

The wealthy households of ancient China had a special room for childbirth called the artemisia room where this plant (also known as mugwort) was burnt to attract kindred spirits and to bring about a state of tranquillity to mother and child.

One of the most highly prized plants of ancient China was the mo-lu-hwa, a species of jasmine; just one bloom has the power to perfume a whole room.

The Greeks owed much of their medicinal and anatomical knowledge to the Egyptians. As in Egypt, aromatics were literally a way of life. Sweet incense was burnt in the temples, city squares and during state ceremonies. Many homes were equipped with an altar called a *thyterion* on which incense was burnt to appease the gods.

It seems the Greeks were not satisfied with perfuming their clothes and their bodies: food and wine had to be scented as well. Rose, violet and even myrrh-scented wines were regarded as nothing short of celebrational nectar. However, they had an ulterior motive: perfume, particularly rose, was believed to quell the intoxicating effects of alcohol, which meant they could drink more! (Indeed, rose oil is known to have a specific healing effect on the liver.)

Hippocrates extolled the virtues of a daily aromatic bath and scented massage to prolong life. In fact, massage with aromatic oils was deemed so efficacious that Plato is said to have reproached Herodicus (one of the teachers of Hippocrates) for protracting the miserable existence of the aged!

The Romans spent vast sums on aromatics and on their elaborate public baths – an idea adopted from the Egyptians. Wealthy families would while away their days at the baths being massaged with aromatic oils by the unfortunate eunuch slave whose sole function in life was to knead and pummel his master.

The Arabs were explorers of some renown. They travelled by sea and by land to distant countries in search of aromatics and artefacts. Arab coins have been found in as far away places as Russia, Germany and Sweden! From their travels in the Far East, they brought back many potent aromatics which included sandalwood, cassia, camphor, nutmeg, myrrh and cloves. These aromatics were used in both perfumery and medicine.

Physicians harnessed the powerful germicidal properties of essential oils by disinfecting their bodies and their clothes with a pleasing mixture of sandalwood, camphor and rosewater. Not only did this protect them from infection, it served to create a perfumed persona to cheer the sick. This practice was also advocated by Hippocrates, the 'father of medicine', several centuries before.

By the eleventh century, the famous Arabian physician/philosopher/mathematician/astronomer Abu Ibn Sina (known as Avicenna in the West) had perfected the art of distillation to capture the volatile essences from plants. So advanced was his method, that the apparatus for distillation has altered very little in 900 years. He also used massage, traction (for broken limbs) and a detoxifying all-fruit diet as part of his healing regime.

By the twelfth century, perfumes of Arabia were famous throughout Europe. The crusading Knights brought back with them not only exotic and costly perfumes, but the knowledge of how to distil them.

Mediaeval herbals contain references to lavender water and many methods of using essential oils, even though some of the moralists and religious leaders regarded the practice as frivolous and even immoral. The women of British households were skilled in making herbal medicines and pomanders for scenting linen and warding off fleas and moths. Some of the wealthy homes even installed their own still for extracting essential oils from plants to be used in medicine and perfumery. Incidentally, it is a well-documented fact that perfumers (who, of course, were pervaded by essential oils) were often immune to the plague.

The Norman conquest brought with it, among many other customs, the strewing on floors of aromatic plants that gave off their scent when walked upon. The insecticidal and bactericidal properties of aromatic plants helped ward off disease by killing air-borne bacteria and deterring fleas and lice. People smothered their unwashed bodies and clothes with perfume and carried little bouquets of aromatic herbs (tussie mussies) with them to prevent infectious illness and to mask the stench of the filthy streets.

By the seventeenth century, the use of herbs and essential oils in medicine saw a decline in favour of the newly emerging chemical drugs. Some of these, particularly mercury, proved to be horrifyingly dangerous. In her book *Green Pharmacy* Barbara Griggs describes some of the grotesque side-effects of mercury which was administered as a cure for syphilis. In retrospect, dying of the disease itself would seem infinitely preferable to the agonies of death from mercury poisoning.

By the nineteenth century, as today, chemists were intent on sifting out the so-called impurities of plants in order to isolate their 'active principles'. However, these 'impurities' are a necessary part of the whole because they work in harmony with the active principle, thus preventing side-effects.

THE TWENTIETH CENTURY PIONEERS

The founder of aromatherapy as we know it was René Gattefossé, a French chemist who worked in his family's perfumery business in the 1920s. At first, his research was confined to the cosmetic uses of essential oils, but he soon realised that many of these oils had powerful antiseptic properties as well. Following a laboratory explosion, his hand was severely burned. He plunged it into a dish of lavender essence and was astonished how quickly the burn healed. There was no sign of infection, nor even scar to remind him of the accident.

This incident led Gattefossé to investigate the use of essential oils in skin conditions and to undertake a great deal of research into their medicinal use. He published a book on the subject in 1928 entitled *Aromatherapie*, thus coining the word which has been used ever since.

A great deal of interest in aromatherapy was kindled in France and Italy as a result of Gattefossé's book. Professor Paolo Rovesti, Director of the Instituto Derivati Vegatali in Milan, demonstrated that smelling oils of certain plants can relieve anxiety states and depression. He used the oils produced from locally grown fruits such as bergamot, orange and lemon. He soaked bits of cotton wool in essential oils and passed it under the noses of his patients. This, he said, helped to evoke and release suppressed memories and emotions that were having a detrimental effect on the health of these people.

Dr Jean Valnet, a French doctor and ex-army surgeon, has contributed most to the medical assessment and acceptance of the treatment. Valnet used essential oils for the wounds and burns of soldiers during the Second World War. Later, in his book *Aromatherapie*, he describes how he successfully treated several long-term psychiatric patients with essential oils. These people also had physical symptoms caused by the side-effects of the drugs they had been given to control their depression and hallucinations. They were gradually weaned off the drugs and Valnet treated them with internal doses of essential oils instead. Both physical and mental symptoms were relieved, sometimes within days of discontinuing the drugs. The English translation of this book *The Practice of Aromatherapy* has become a classic for aromatherapists. Valnet is also the president of the Societé Française de Phytotherapie et d'Aromatherapie.

The Austrian born biochemist Marguerite Maury could be hailed as the mother of holistic aromatherapy. Although inspired by Gattefossé, she developed a special massage technique of applying essential oils along the nerve centres of the spine as well as to the face. Mme Maury was not happy with the idea of administering the essences orally. She also introduced the idea of the individual prescription whereby oils were chosen according to the individual needs of her clients. Her clients (mainly wealthy women seeking rejuvenation) reported dramatic improvement in their skin condition as a result of her treatments. To their amazement, there were also some interesting 'side-effects'; many experienced relief from rheumatic pain, deeper sleep and a generally improved mental state. The effects lasted weeks or sometimes months after treatments had finished.

Marguerite Maury was totally dedicated to her work, and in 1962 and 1967 she was awarded two international prizes for her research into essential oils and cosmetology.

In the English translation from the French of her book entitled *The Secret of Life and Youth* Danièl Ryman – ex-pupil of Mme Maury who has continued her work for over 20 years – writes, 'Marguerite

Maury possessed some of the eccentricities of genius . . . she was a veritable whirlwind of energy and enthusiasm, working ceaselessly until, quite literally, she died of sheer overwork, of a stroke during the night of 25 September, 1968'.

Marguerite Maury was 73 years of age when she died. Her husband and colleague Dr E.A. Maury writes, 'She continues to show the way for those who have been willing to recognise her and will long do so for those who seek a new orientation for their moral and physical well-being'.

Robert Tisserand, a British practising aromatherapist, author and researcher, is the author of one of the first books in English on this hitherto rather elusive (except in France) therapy. In his first book entitled *The Art of Aromatherapy*, he discusses the history and the therapeutic properties and applications of a number of essences. It may be fair to say that this book, perhaps above any other, has generated a great deal of interest, world-wide, in the healing art of aromatherapy.

3

What Aromatherapy Can Do For You

AROMATHERAPY can do a little or a great deal for you, depending on how much effort you are prepared to put into safeguarding your health and increasing your vitality. Are you prepared to give up smoking for instance, or to cut down on the amount of caffeine, alcohol, sugar and junk-food you may consume? How often do you get out for a walk in the countryside or even in the local park? Can you spare as little as half an hour each day to unwind or to commune with nature?

Aromatherapy can help many disorders, but for the best results it should form part of a holistic health regime. By this I mean we should look beyond the symptoms to the cause and to the prevention of illness. It is important to remember that illness does not strike 'out of the blue' even though it may seem that way at times. There are many possible causes of ill health; heredity plays a part (most unfairly) but, in the main, its origin lies in our mental state, life-style and diet.

Holistic aromatherapy, in common with other holistic therapies, demands a great deal of commitment from yourself. It may not be as easy as surrendering your body to the doctor and simply taking the medicine, nor can you expect an over-night cure. However, the long-term results are well worth the effort.

The self-help suggestions as outlined in this book will help to increase your energy levels and restore a sense of harmony to your life, no matter how frenetic that life may be. In all forms of natural therapy, which aim to stimulate rather than to suppress the body's natural defences, the axiom is: by creating favourable conditions in

19

the whole person, body-mind-spirit, the body will heal itself. This is also known as the holistic approach. If this concept is new to you, turn to Chapter 7 where you will find many suggestions for creating harmony at all levels within your being.

WHAT ABOUT PROFESSIONAL AROMATHERAPY TREATMENT?

Should you decide to consult a professional aromatherapist (see the list of professional bodies in the appendix), do not expect exactly the same treatment from every aromatherapist. Individual therapists tend to approach the art in their own unique way. Much will depend on where they were trained and whether they are skilled in other therapies and techniques such as reflexology (pressure point massage of the feet), Touch For Health (muscle testing, a diagnostic technique), medical herbalism, spiritual healing or perhaps nutrition.

A good aromatherapist, whether basically intuitive (akin to a spiritual healer), clinical (advocating internal doses of essential oils) or multi-skilled, will tread the holistic path. A personalised healing programme will be devised to suit your temperament and specific needs. Most importantly, there will be an empathy between yourself and your therapist. For without empathy, very little in the way of *true* healing (of mind-body-spirit) can be achieved (see page 41).

In the following case studies, we will glimpse aromatherapy in action from several different levels: the simple, almost symptomatic approach (which does occasionally have a role to play); the holistic/intuitive (valuable for those suffering from stress-related problems), and finally, clinical/holistic – the ultimate that can be achieved in holistic healing.

SOME CASE STUDIES

Scabies

Scabies is a skin disease caused by infestation with the parasitic 'itch mite' (*Sarcoptes Scabei*). The mite can be caught from farm animals – particularly sheep.

Elizabeth: Elizabeth, a young woman who lives with her sister in a remote and primitive cottage in the Welsh mountains, came to see me about an infestation of scabies. Her lower back and abdomen were badly infected. Due to frantic scratching, the skin had become very inflamed. It was also covered with watery blisters caused by the burrowing of the itch mites.

Elizabeth was prepared to put her trust in essential oils rather than resort to an even stronger preparation from her doctor who had already prescribed an ointment which had not worked.

First I advised her to take four to six garlic capsules a day for the duration of the treatment which we hoped would not be too prolonged. No matter what the advertisements say to the contrary, garlic is always perceptible on the breath, even when it is taken in capsule form. As much of the the sulphurous pungency of garlic is also eliminated through the skin, it occurred to me that it might succeed in gassing the squatters out! Furthermore, sulphur-based ointments are used in orthodox treatments for scabies. Next I gave her some lavender essence to put in the bath (a tin bath in front of the kitchen range). Then I 'doctored' some ready-made beeswax ointment with essences of lavender and peppermint which I advised Elizabeth to apply liberally, two or three times a day. The doctor had already advised Elizabeth to boil her bed linen and not to share any of her clothes with her sister – scabies is very infectious.

A week later, Elizabeth was pleased to report that the itching had stopped. The inflammation gradually calmed down, and within three weeks, her skin had healed, though it was very flaky. I gave her a jar of home-made skin cream containing almond oil, cocoa butter and rosewater to soften her skin.

Athlete's Foot

Athlete's foot (*Tinea pedis*) is a fungal infection of the skin between the toes. It may also appear on other parts of the body in the form of an itchy rash known as ringworm. Excessive perspiration in poorly ventilated footwear invites infection which can also be picked up in the changing rooms of public swimming pools or sports centres. Severe cases of athlete's foot, involving the toenails and other areas of the foot (fissured heels is a symptom) is usually indicative of a poor state of health in general and needs to be treated holistically.

A course of vitamin B-complex and dietary reform may need to be implemented.

Howard: Howard is a keen walker, spending much of his spare time climbing in the hills and tramping through mud and running streams. His feet are usually cocooned in two pairs of thick socks and heavy walking boots – even during hot weather! No wonder his feet perspire profusely and are prone to athlete's foot.

When Howard first showed me his feet, they were in a sorry state. Apart from the sore cracks between most of his toes, the skin was heavily calloused and his heels were covered in blisters (he had just returned from a particularly arduous walk). Howard had tried all the proprietary athlete's foot remedies, but found they were only partially effective; the infection would always return with a vengeance within a few days of discontinuing with the ointment or powder.

My first suggestion was sunlight, fresh air and scrupulous hygiene – and to keep the feet as dry as possible. Howard realised the importance of avoiding walking barefoot in public places such as swimming pools or on other people's carpets, so he decided to walk barefoot on grass and on the beach whenever possible, or simply to sit outside and expose his feet to the elements.

I gave Howard some lavender essence to apply neat (one or two drops) to the fissures between his toes, three times a day. Much to his surprise, the oil did not sting. Lavender, in common with most essential oils, is kind to sore, grazed or infected skin. Within days, the skin had healed. Howard has now become scrupulous about washing his socks in fairly hot soapy water (they cannot be washed in extremely hot water because he favours woollen socks, though cotton would be preferable) and regularly airing his boots. He also puts a couple of drops of lavender essence on the toe-end of his socks as a preventative measure.

A year later, during the unusually hot summer of 1990, he developed a minor break-out which lavender cleared up within a day or two. The only side-effect reported: the sweetest smelling boots known to man!

Pre-Menstrual Tension

This condition is more aptly termed pre-menstrual syndrome (PMS) because tension is just one of a number of other emotional and physical disturbances experienced by women a few days (or two weeks) before the onset of menstruation. Before we look at the case study of Anna, I would like to put forward my own views about PMS.

Anthropologists have commented on the fact that women in primitive communities rarely experience menstrual problems. Not because they may relate more positively to menstruation and to their sexuality (as some psychologists have suggested), but more likely, I believe, because they rarely have the opportunity to experience menstruation. During their fertile years they are either pregnant or breastfeeding. Breastfeeding can delay the onset of menstruation for three years. Could it be that a *degree* of PMS (I do not mean suicidal or murderous tendencies) is a perfectly reasonable response by a healthy reproductive system to the unnatural state of non-pregnancy? Of course, I am not suggesting that women should give in to biology (perish the thought), but that PMS is not quite the pathological state that a few health experts would appear to be suggesting.

Certainly, it is true that PMS is exacerbated by stress and a poor diet (which is why it can be remedied to a great extent), but the real culprit is fluid retention – caused by natural changes in body chemistry.

Anna: Anna telephoned early one morning in a distressed state, hoping I would be able to see her that day. I called several hours later, by which time she had calmed down a little, but was smoking one cigarette after another.

Anna was 38 at the time, a single parent with an 11-year-old daughter. She managed to hold down a job as a journalist with a local newspaper, but was finding it increasingly difficult to produce a reasonable standard of work when suffering from PMS, which was sometimes debilitating. The symptoms she endured varied from month to month, worsening or improving according to the circumstances of her life at the time.

On this particular occasion, Anna was suffering from anxiety and insomnia, spotty skin, bloating (her abdomen had swollen alarmingly) and a craving for sweet food – particularly chocolate. We sat talking for about an hour while Anna tearfully related how she had recently been 'ditched' by her lover (a young man of 23) for a girl of 18. She had reason to be depressed this time.

Anna chose essences of ylang-ylang (her favourite), bergamot and geranium from a selection of possibles set out before her. Although ylang-ylang is generally regarded as an aphrodisiac oil in aromatherapy, not a good choice in the circumstances one might have thought, she took an instant dislike to the less interesting herbal essences. She particularly disliked marjoram – an essence used for grief, said to be an *anti*-aphrodisiac. However, I always allow the person to trust their own instincts in such matters. Geranium though was obviously a good choice because of its diuretic properties – and bergamot for its cheerful and uplifting aroma. Both essences blend well with ylang-ylang and have a balancing affect on the central nervous system.

The treatment consisted of a full-body massage, with particular attention to her back (the area either side of the spine is the gateway to the entire nervous system). I also worked on balancing the energies within her aura (see page 39).

By the end of the treatment, Anna was almost asleep – I left her alone to enjoy quietly the experience of newfound peace. Later she phoned to tell me how much lighter she felt, as if a burden had somehow been lifted from her shoulders.

For about a year afterwards Anna received aromatherapy massage whenever she felt the need – once, sometimes twice, a month. We worked together on gradually improving her diet. When she remembered, she also took an evening primrose oil supplement specially formulated for PMS. She had been in the habit of drinking five or six mugs of coffee a day (a massive onslaught to the nervous system). Eventually, we reached the stage where she could avoid it altogether a few days before a period, but she continued to drink one or two small cups a day at other times. As for smoking, we reached a compromise. She felt she could not give up totally, but settled for three or four slim cigars a day instead of ten to fifteen cigarettes.

Anna uses essential oils in her bath as well as for skin-care and as perfume to uplift her spirits. She has developed a passion for a blend of ylang-ylang and patchouli.

Although Anna still experiences slight bloating and feels a little weepy before a period, her energy levels in general have increased. She sleeps more soundly and is able to think more clearly.

Several months ago Anna and her daughter moved to the South East of England. The last time I heard from her she was planning to marry her live-in partner – they have been running a wholefood shop and café!

Grief

The following case study is unusual because Charlotte (not her real name) had not revealed to me the *actual* reason why she felt the need for aromatherapy. Instead, much of the truth came to me intuitively and was later verified, quite by chance, by a friend of Charlotte.

This study also serves to illustrate the very real need for what is known in healing circles as 'psychic protection'. Uncomfortable feelings absorbed from those who seek our help (and that includes simply offering a sympathetic ear), can linger for many hours or even days – unless we learn how to dissipate such feelings. This could be by employing techniques such as 'auric control', 'nature attunement', or simply by taking a shower and a dose of Dr Bach's Rescue Remedy (see page 121).

Charlotte: Charlotte is a wealthy woman in her early forties who views aromatherapy as nothing more than an upmarket beauty treatment. She booked herself in for the works as she put it – a facial and full-body massage. She felt she needed a little pampering.

This is all I shall relate about Charlotte's circumstances in order to protect her anonymity, but suffice it to say, I decided to play along with her idea of aromatherapy being simply a pleasant way to relax – indeed, you do not need to be ill to enjoy the benefits of aromatherapy massage.

My first impression of Charlotte was that she was pleasant enough, but I sensed a very private person under the rather theatrical facade. For her massage, she chose a blend of frankincense, rose and cedarwood. She began to relax into the massage almost immediately. The atmosphere of the room was enhanced by the gentle background sounds of reed pipes. The music, combined with the aroma of the oils, began to lull me (I am not sure about Charlotte!) into a meditative state. Although I had not intended to work on her aura, my hands began to scan the energy field surrounding her physical body. As I moved over the 'heart centre' I experienced a heaviness in my chest. Charlotte coughed. I felt she was holding back, refusing to release the pain which weighed heavily on her heart.

At the end of the treatment, Charlotte showed no signs of distress. In fact, she said she felt wonderful, and booked another appointment for the following week.

That night I could not sleep. The night after that my sleep was invaded by a series of disturbing dreams. Foolishly, I had not bothered to carry out any of the psychic protective techniques I had been taught as a 'probationer healer' at a school of esoteric studies. I had convinced myself that the massage had been no more than superficial.

To cut this story short, for several more aromatherapy sessions with Charlotte, I experienced what I came to recognise as grief. However, I had learned to shake off any lingering discomfort quite easily after the initial shock to my psyche.

Charlotte continued with the aromatherapy treatments for several months (once every three to four weeks). She used essential oils in her bath and to perfume rooms. The essences she chose tended to be of the wood or resinous families – sandalwood, cedarwood, frankincense and myrrh, heightened with rose or ylang-ylang, occasionally clary-sage.

After about the fourth or fifth month into the course of treatments, I began to feel a lessening of the pain, but not once had she confided that anything was wrong. It was also at about this time that a friend of Charlotte (whom I met at a party) commented on how much better Charlotte was looking – considering the circumstances.

'Of course, she must live with the tragedy of her daughter's suicide for the rest of her life . . .'

Hyperactivity

A wayward child, forever up to mischief and straining at the bit to dash around, is not necessarily hyperactive. The truly hyperactive child sleeps very little (possibly only four to five hours a night), has an attention span obviously shorter than other children and behaves in a way that is chaotic rather than simply energetic. Teachers and parents, of course, are driven to distraction.

Many of these children are put on drugs to help control their behaviour. A drastic step in most cases, because much can be done to reduce hyperactive behaviour safely and, I believe, more humanely.

The first step is diet. One of the pioneers in this field is Dr Ben Feingold who, in the 1960s, was the head of the allergy department at the Kaiser-Permanente Medical Centre in San Francisco, California. He found that hyperactive children improved dramatically on a diet which excluded all artificially flavoured and coloured foods. Hyperactive children (and some adults as well) were observed suddenly to outgrow behaviour problems along with their skin allergies.

The following study of Owen may perhaps be regarded as only a partial success. As is most common in holistic healing, too few people are prepared to stick to the dietary disciplines for long. This is largely due to social pressures. It is extremely difficult to wean a child off junk-food, especially when his or her friends are allowed to indulge – with seemingly no ill effects. The stress of being a 'social outcast' may outweigh some of the benefits of a totally pure, wholefood diet, so it is often necessary come to a compromise over such matters, as Owen's parents decided to do.

Owen: When I first met Owen he was seven years old – a whirlwind of a boy, tearing around the house, yelling at the top of his voice. Many children of his age are boisterous, but Owen was disruptive. His parents, Bronwen and David, were in despair. They had received yet another letter from the school complaining about Owen's lack of attention in class and his bullying of other children.

Even though Owen was intelligent (he could impress his teachers on occasions), he was generally regarded as a 'problem child' with special needs. He slept very lightly (awakening at the slightest sound) and for no more than six hours a night (if his parents were lucky). Most seven year olds sleep for about ten hours at a stretch.

Bronwen explained that her son had been difficult from day one, crying most of the day and night, demanding constant attention. Needless to say, Bronwen and David were exhausted. In fact, I first found out about Owen because I was treating Bronwen and David for 'stress'. Although the aromatherapy massage was helping to buffer some of the strain, it was obvious to us all that Owen needed help as well.

It was agreed that I should see Owen on his home ground in order to assess his true behaviour. Owen was keen to show me his new electric racing car set and let me by the arm to his room. I was taken aback by the decor – vivid red, yellow and green geometric patterns screaming from every wall. Surely a most inappropriate colour scheme for the bedroom of a hyperactive child? The patterns appeared to jump into the room! I did not have the nerve to mention this to Owen's parents – a failing on my part.

Owen's diet was appalling. Although he would eat foods such as salads, fresh fruit and wholemeal bread (not always the case with hyperactive children), he was also allowed to eat far too many sweets and chocolate bars washed down with cola, squash and tea. In fact, Bronwen had already discovered that Owen would 'go berserk' after a tin of soup containing monosodium glutamate, or fish fingers coloured with tartrazine (now largely withdrawn as a food colouring agent).

I gave Owen's parents the address of the Hyperactive Children's Support Group (HACSG) and suggested they write off for the HACSG diet sheet (based on the Feingold diet).

I mixed a massage oil containing lavender and clary-sage, and asked Owen if he liked the aroma. He approved straight away. We were doubtful as to whether Owen would lie still long enough for a back massage, but he surprised us by putting up with it for about ten minutes. In fact, after the first few minutes of wriggling and giggling, he began to enjoy it. Owen knew his parents had been having aromatherapy massage, so I think it made him feel grown-up and important.

Bronwen reported the next day that Owen had slept deeply for about six hours, and for the first time in ages had not woken up several times during the night to go to the toilet.

Owen received aromatherapy massage weekly for about three months. He also took a nightly bath containing lavender, clary-sage or chamomile – sometimes a blend of all three essences. I prescribed the Bach Flower Remedies (completely harmless 'vibrational' remedies, see page 121) to help transmute his sometimes angry and violent behaviour into positive energy.

His parents half-heartedly attempted to implement the HACSG diet and applied evening primrose oil to Owen's skin (as recommended by the HACSG).

Certainly the massage and energy balancing (of the aura) worked wonders – he always slept deeply afterwards. However, the effect did not last for more than two days at a time because Owen's diet was still too high in white sugar and chemical additives. I taught

Bronwen and David the back massage sequence to use as a 'first-aid' measure. Aromatic bathing and massage became a nightly ritual which had to be carried out before Owen would go to bed.

Owen's behaviour did, in fact, improve enough for it to be noticed at school. However, I was not entirely happy with the situation because aromatherapy was being used mainly as a palliative. Therefore, I suggested homoeopathy which I hoped would go deeper. The homoeópath was happy to allow Owen to continue enjoying the aromatic baths and massage, but was less concerned about diet – some homoeopaths do not advocate dietary reform.

This, of course, suited Owen and his parents. Only time will tell if homoeopathic treatment has been successful.

Aids

Karin Cutter is a naturopathic doctor practising in New South Wales, Australia. I am most grateful to her for allowing me to use this remarkable case study of John.[4] Here is an extract from her letter:

John has always gone out of his way to try and persuade similar sufferers that there may be help for them in alternative therapies. Unfortunately, few of them are interested or want to stick to the dietary disciplines for long. Neither John nor I have any objection to use of his history, especially if the information is of benefit to someone else.

John: In 1985, John had to give up his career as a consulting engineer because he was desperately ill. He was transferred to a hospital in Sydney where he was told he had AIDS. The doctors gave him two years to live.

However, John was not prepared to die. He found an holistic therapist who taught him about dietary reform, meditation and visualisation. Despite the hospital specialist's scepticism, he began to show signs of recovery. His energy levels increased and the walnut-sized swellings in his neck and groin began to shrink. But in December 1985, John suffered a setback. He developed an allergy to a powerful, broad-spectrum antibiotic he had been given to treat an attack of bronchitis. He lost a lot of weight and the purple-black lesions on his skin (a tell-tale symptom of AIDS) began to spread. He also suffered bouts of depression and confusion. The doctors rated his chances as virtually nil.

Even though he could barely stand, John made one last desperate bid for survival. He contacted the naturopathic clinic where Karin Cutter was based (his original naturopath had moved to Melbourne). John was the clinic's first ever AIDS patient.

Treatment was geared to boosting John's immune system which was being battered by various systemic fungi and intestinal parasites. First of all he was put on a yeast-free, sugar-free diet and treated with essential oils of garlic, tea-tree and thyme. In fact, tea-tree, with its myriad of uses, proved to be the most helpful. The oil was employed in various ways which included baths, steam inhalations and suppositories. When external treatment with tea-tree no longer produced any improvement (after many months), the oil was given by mouth which resulted in further elimination of toxins.

John's recovery attracted a great deal of media attention in Australia. It is now five years since the date of his official death sentence. He is alive and well, devoting much of his time to encouraging and supporting other AIDS sufferers in their quest for life.

Important: Karin Cutter would like to point out that if you have AIDS, or indeed any other serious illness, do not 'give it a go' on your own. Do seek the guidance of a qualified and accredited practitioner – holistic or orthodox. Without a true understanding of the underlying nature of your illness, the consequences could be devastating.

AND MUCH MORE . . .

The six case studies included in this book are all that space would allow. Volumes could be written about the men, women and children (and animals too) who have been helped by essential oils in some way.

Clinical aromatherapists are increasingly employing essential oils to help serious diseases. Ellen Asjes, from Holland, for example, is a qualified physiotherapist and *hielpraktiker* (equivalent to a US naturopathic doctor). Ellen has successfuly treated her husband Ray Smith for cancer of the liver. Essential oils played an important role in his recovery. She has also helped a man diagnosed as carrying AIDS antibodies in his blood (HIV positive). After treatment (which included essential oils), blood and urine tests showed that HIV was no longer present.

Although *intuitive* aromatherapy is much derided by orthodox practitioners (and even by a few scientifically minded aromatherapists), it too has its place in the holistic scheme of things. Counselling, an important part of intuitive aromatherapy, and healing massage may be instrumental in nipping the disease process in the bud, as it were. It is increasingly recognised (even in orthodox circles) that unhappiness or 'stress' is a contributing factor in the development of chronic illness.

4

How Does It Work?

IN SIMPLISTIC TERMS, aromatherapy works by influencing at least two levels simultaneously: the physical and the emotional. We could include another level – the spiritual. Although we may perceive these levels as separate, they are in fact interrelated – we cannot in reality separate the parts that make up the whole.

Although the mind-body effects of essences can be verified by science, the spiritual dimension is, of course, elusive – as ethereal as the fragrance of a beautiful flower. Be that as it may, I shall attempt to explain the spiritual aspect in my own terms. First though, let us explore the more tangible routes an essential oil may take on its sojourn through mind-body.

SKIN ABSORPTION

Many people believe that the skin is an impervious covering, the sole function of which is to keep the blood and organs in and water out. To suggest to them that the skin is capable of absorbing essential oils by diffusing them across the fine blood capillaries (under the surface of the skin) and into the main bloodstream is bound to meet with a certain amount of scepticism, if not ridicule.

It is true that water and watery substances cannot be absorbed into the bloodstream through the skin, although the upper layers will temporarily hold a little water. This is noticeable after a long soak in the bath; the pads of your fingertips will take on a wrinkled appearance. However, René Gattefossé, the father of aromatherapy, established without a doubt that the skin can absorb fatty substances, provided that their molecular structure is small enough.

Interestingly, the black witches of antiquity used poisonous ointments impregnated with extracts of hemlock, belladonna and other lethal plants, to see off their enemies. Up until the early twentieth century syphilis was treated by rubbing in mercury ointment. It was very difficult to judge the amount absorbed, resulting in some horrible side-effects, though the infection was often eradicated. Administering drugs by inunction (through the skin) has been made safer recently with the introduction of a measured dose. For example oestrogen and trinitrin have been administered in a patch applied to the skin.

In skin absorption, it is thought that the essential oils, with their very fine aromatic molecules, pass through the hair follicles, which contain sebum, an oily liquid with which the essential oils have an affinity. From here the oils diffuse into the bloodstream or are taken up by the lymph and interstitial fluid (a liquid surrounding all body cells) to other parts of the body.

If the skin is healthy, it takes only a few minutes for the molecules to be absorbed; much longer if the skin is congested or if there is much subcutaneous fat. The skin cannot, however, absorb essential oils if it is perspiring – after a sauna for instance. You will need to wait several hours before applying the oils. A few minutes' facial sauna, however, is fine because it warms the skin just enough to facilitate absorption. People with congested skin often benefit from aromatic baths (if not too hot) and full-body massage because the skin of the abdomen, inner thighs and upper arms is much softer and therefore more capable of absorption.

Once in the bloodstream, the aromatic molecules affect the body in a similar way to herbal medicine. Some have an affinity with the kidneys for instance (juniper, cypress), others may influence the hormones via the adrenal cortex (geranium, basil) or, as mentioned in Chapter 1, they may have a 'normalising' effect on both mind and body (bergamot, geranium).

Even though essential oils are sometimes given orally (especially in the case of garlic) they can often be even more effective when applied to the skin. This can also be seen with evening primrose oil; though not an essential oil, it appears to work better when applied externally for the treatment of hyperactivity in children.

Oral doses are not always successful because absorption from the gut is often impaired in these children. Incidentally, vitamins were applied percutaneously to treat severely vitamin-deficient ex-prisoners too ill to take them by mouth after the Second World War.

ABSORPTION VIA THE LUNGS

When inhaled, the aromatic molecules of essential oils reach the lungs from where they diffuse across the air sacs into the surrounding blood capillaries (which lie just under the surface of the sacs) and eventually find their way into the main blood vessels from where they circulate in the blood and exert their therapeutic effect.

The detrimental effect of some odours such as toxic industrial wastes, and the results of snorting cocaine, or of solvent sniffing, is proof enough that odours, beneficial or otherwise, do enter the body as gases and can alter our physical and mental health.

THE SENSE OF SMELL AND THE MIND

Just how odours are perceived is a complicated and as yet not fully understood process. The following explanation is the generally accepted current theory. Odoriferous substances, such as essential oils, throw off molecules which are detected by the olfactory cells in the upper part of the nose. These cells are specialized sensory neurones embedded in a mucous membrane, each of which connects directly with the brain by means of a single long nerve fibre. Each cell body has a rod-like extension to the surface of the membrane, terminating in a brush of hair-like structures which are super-sensitive. Before an aromatic molecule can be detected, it must first be dissolved in the mucus. Responses to the aromatic molecule are then sent in the form of impulses via the nerve fibres to the olfactory area in the brain. Because the sensory processes ('hairs') are in *direct* contact with the source of smell, and because the olfactory cells connect *directly* with the brain, the sense of smell has a powerful and immediate effect.

This is because the area of the brain associated with smell is very closely connected with the limbic area of the brain which is concerned with our most subtle responses such as emotion, memory, sex-drive and intuition. The olfactory area of the brain also connects with the hypothalamus, a very important structure which controls the entire hormonal system by influencing the 'master gland' itself – the pituitary.

From this, we may conclude that any process which can send impulses directly to the brain can be used to influence the physical body and the emotions. For example, the aroma of hot food, especially when flavoured with herbs or spices, will stimulate the appetite by making one's mouth water and causing the digestive juices to flow.

Aroma, like music, can often evoke memories. Some people only have to take the faintest whiff of the entrance hall of a hospital to be sharply transported back in time to relive a traumatic hospital experience (endured during childhood perhaps); they may feel shaky or even nauseous. Other aromas conjure up pleasant memories of first love perhaps, or possibly a visit to a well-loved grandmother who always smelled of lavender-water. Interestingly, scientists are now saying that odour is different in *degree* to memory rather than different in kind.[5]

Critics of aromatherapy have pointed out that the sense of smell becomes quickly exhausted as the olfactory cells in the nose soon become saturated and cease to detect the aroma, so the effects of aromatherapy can only be short-lived. However, as Marguerite Maury and other eminent people in the field of aromatherapy have discovered, the emotional (as well as the physical) effects can last for sometime afterwards, whether the aroma is still perceptible or not.

For those who prefer scientific evidence for the effects of essential oils on the mind, let me draw your attention to some experiments carried out in the last ten years by John Steele (an American research worker) and Maxwell Cade, a British biophysicist. Volunteers were wired up to an EEG (electroencephalograph) machine called a 'Mind Mirror' which records brainwave patterns.

They observed the effects on the mind of inhaling various essential oils on cotton wool. Those essences which are known to stimulate clarity of thought (rosemary, basil, peppermint) produced more beta brainwaves indicating a state of mental alertness. Some of the floral anti-depressants such as rose and neroli induced more alpha, theta and delta waves, indicating a quietening of mental 'chatter' and the mind moving into a state approaching meditation.

At Warwick University (England), doctors Steve Van Toller and George Dodd have been carrying out a great deal of research in recent years into the relationship between smell and emotion. Although they have tended to experiment with synthetic perfumes and other odoriferous substances apart from essential oils, their findings are very interesting from an aromatherapy viewpoint. They have been able to prove without doubt that aroma has a profound influence on mind and body. Aromatherapists now have the weight of scientific evidence to drop on the die-hard sceptics who delight in ridiculing the 'airy-faerie' practice of aromatherapy.

Among the many experiments carried out at Warwick, there is one of particular note: the discovery that skin can respond to odours – even those we cannot smell. One substance used was the sex pheromone excreted in the urine of the boar. Surprisingly, many people have a *specific anosmia* to the pheromone (they cannot smell it) even though their sense of smell in other respects may be normal.

Volunteers were wired up to an EEG machine which records skin responses as well as brainwave patterns. Very clear skin responses to the pheromone were recorded – even in those who said they could not detect the odour. Those who could smell the pheromone either loved it or hated it.

It was also discovered at Warwick that, if we dislike an aroma, we are able to block its effect on the central nervous system. This supports the case for using the oils we like best, especially for stress-related problems.

The pheromone experiment puts me in mind of the effects of sandalwood essence: people can sometimes have a specific anosmia to its aroma. Most people though, find the aroma extremely tenacious. A few find it repugnant, detecting a 'sweaty' note. Others find the aroma adorable and can testify to its potent aphrodisiac affect. Furthermore, as in the pheromone experiment, either sex may respond favourably to sandalwood's seductive aroma; or conversely, respond with an 'ugh!' Somehow, sandalwood oil must be hermaphroditic in nature!

Another mystifying mind-body phenomenon is auto-suggestion. Some years ago, as a student of aromatherapy at my first workshop, I encountered the captivating aroma of sandalwood. Having put down the bottle, but still entranced by the (to my nose at any rate) sweet, dulcet tones of the essence, I decided to take another whiff to convince myself I had not really been dreaming. Yes, it was truly divine. However, as I replaced the cap, to my utter amazement, I noticed it was labelled 'Geranium' – I had picked up the wrong bottle. Anyone familiar with the clear, highly distinctive aroma of geranium would know that one would need to be totally anosmic to confuse it with the soft, deep notes of sandalwood. Needless to say, as soon as I realised my error, the spell had been broken: the piercing aroma of geranium came through shrill and clear. Now, what would an EEG machine have made of that? Incidentally, I have never since been able to work such magic!

AROMA PREFERENCE

People, as well as animals, secrete substances called pheromones which are responsible for their own individual body scent. No two people smell exactly alike – though there are similarities between races. This may be partly due to the type of food eaten. People who like spicy food for example, also plump for strong, penetrating essences such as patchouli and ginger. High dairy food consumers prefer light floral fragrances.

Aroma preference is also largely influenced by our body odour. Emotions, illness, the pill (and other drugs) as well as hormonal changes such as puberty, pregnancy and the menopause all influence body odour and our aroma preferences. This explains why the same perfume smells different on each person and why we go off certain essential oils, and begin to enjoy the ones previously distasteful to us. As we grow older, our bodies secrete different pheromones, and consequently a favourite perfume of our youth may seem totally obnoxious to us in maturity.

While on the subject of body odour, during the sixteenth century, valerian was a popular perfume. To the modern nose, it stinks. However, it would have harmonised nicely with the bodily secretions (excretions?) of the infrequently washed bodies of the era.

Aroma conditioning or 'fashion' may also play a part in aroma preference. This is a pity because this kind of 'brain-washing' inhibits personal expression as well as hindering any beneficial mind-body effects of essential oils (because we can 'block' the effect, as mentioned earlier). True, essential oils do not smell like commercial, highly synthetic formulae; but once weaned onto naturals and drawn into the healing aura of essential oils, you will never again fall for the charms of the latest 'Henry' or crave a fix of 'Venom' nor even be allured by an 'Evening in Paradise'!

In aromatherapy, the axiom is: always be guided by your aroma preference. We are instinctively drawn to the essential oil which may be right for our physical and emotional needs at the time.

AROMA AND VIBRATION

Just because the human ear is 'deaf' to high frequency and low frequency sounds, as every scientist knows, it does not mean they do not exist, nor that we cannot be affected by them. Likewise, we can respond to highly diluted fragrances even though we may not be able to smell them (these are conclusions drawn from the results of other experiments carried out at Warwick). This same principle is at work in homoeopathic and Bach Flower remedies. Only the *vibration* or energy pattern of the original medicinal material is actually present in the lactose tablet (homoeopathy) or in the liquid (Bach Flowers). Yet, if the correct remedy is chosen (usually by a skilful and sensitive therapist), the healing effect can be remarkable – and I can testify to this. At this level, we are dealing with vibration, energy – call it what you will. When we take a Bach Flower or homoeopathic remedy, or even when we smell the fragrance of a beautiful flower, the healing effect is triggered at a subtle level, in the auric body (explained below) and filters 'inwards' as it were, to the physical body. Material medicines such as herbs and drugs, move 'outwards' from the physical level, eventually affecting the aura.

This is actually an over-simplification because there is no true separation of mind-body-spirit. We might say we perceive them as separate because they vibrate at different frequencies. All matter and energy is a manifestation of the same thing. Perhaps it may be easier to understand this concept if we consider that matter (from a crystal to a human being) is composed of atoms and sub-atomic particles. Therefore, at this level, according to physics, matter is vibration. Vibration is generally accepted as being another word for energy. Life is essentially energy – so we return to the idea that ALL is ONE.

Where do essential oils fit into this picture? They could be seen as a bridge forming an almost tangible link between the 'two worlds' of spirit and matter. With essential oils we have not only the material substance of the oil with its therapeutic properties, we also have the ethereal aroma, which, according to psychic healers, influences not only the emotions, but also the spiritual aspect. Could fragrance be vibrating at a similar frequency to that of spirit? If so, this would explain why essential oils may influence the spirit directly. It is a law of physics that like attracts like, a principle which is also known in science as *resonance*.

THE AURA

The aura is the radiant life-force surrounding all living and so-called non-living substances of the Earth, such as water and rocks. Before we go any further, the idea of the unity of all things, whether living or non-living is embraced by the relatively new science of quantum physics. In his book *The Tao of Physics* Dr Fritjof Capra explores this concept in depth and comes to the conclusion that eastern mysticism equates well with recent developments in subatomic physics.

The word 'aura' is derived from the Greek *avra* meaning breeze because it is said to be continually in motion. Psychics describe the aura as a rainbow emanation radiating half a metre or more around the body, more or less ovoid in shape. It shimmers and alters in colour depending on our thoughts, emotions and physical state. Muddy colours in the aura indicate negative emotions or ill health; clear colours are generally a positive sign. Some healers (especially acupuncturists) are even able to smell the aura – and this is quite apart from a person's usual body odour.

Although psychics describe the aura differently (according to their own level of psychic perception), it is generally agreed that the aura is composed of at least three layers or levels. These levels vibrate at different frequencies. The physical body or matter vibrates at the slowest or densest frequency; the subtle body, like electricity, vibrates much faster and for this reason we are usually unaware of its existence. The first part of the subtle body or aura is called the *etheric* or *vital* body which emanates about 2.5 centimetres from the physical body; the astral body radiates about 30 centimetres or more around the body; and the mental or spiritual body, which can widen or contract, sometimes extends for metres when we are feeling jubilant or when we are in love, for instance.

The function of the etheric body is to receive and transmit energy or life-force (prana) from the air we breathe. This part of the subtle body can be photographed by a high voltage technique called Kirlian photography. The information captured shows a kind of luminescence and streams of energy flowing from the fingers or toes. To the trained eye, these patterns reflect the emotional and physical state of the individual and can be used as a diagnostic tool.

The astral body, also known as the emotional body, reflects most of the auric colouring. Psychics can often see the auras of women more clearly, possibly because women tend to express their emotions more easily than the average man.

The mental or spiritual body retains all the potential of the individual for his or her future development. It is important to realise however, that all four bodies (which includes the physical) interpenetrate with one another; whatever affects one aspect will affect the whole.

Many of you will choose to dismiss this idea completely out of hand; others may be more open minded. To the former, I suggest you read *The Rainment of Light* by David Tansley and to the others that you try out the following experiment.

To see the aura requires a certain amount of esoteric training (unless you are a natural sensitive), but most people can *feel* it to a greater or lesser degree.

Find yourself a willing partner and sit facing each other. Both of you need to hold out your hands in front and turn the right palm downwards and the left palm upwards. Keep them in this position and place them against the hands of your partner so that you are in physical contact (See Fig. 1). Close your eyes, relax and become aware of your partner's hands; feel the warmth of his or her body. When you feel ready, both of you need to raise your right hand above the other's upturned left hand, but it should remain loose and relaxed, not held stiffly because you will reduce any sensitivity. Stay there for a few minutes and you will begin to experience one of several sensations: it may be a slight breeze, or perhaps a tingling sensation, heat (especially in the palms), static or even a magnetic pull. See how far away you can move your hands from each other and still experience the sensation. Move your hands back and forth or in circles (as if polishing a table) but keep your hands loose and relaxed. You may feel a curious pulling-away sensation or friction.

To break contact, move your hands close together again, slide them away and give them a good shake to remove any tingling (or even tension) picked up from your partner.

The purpose of this exercise is to demonstrate that energy does radiate from the body and that there is more to the human being than guts, blood and bone. Our hands are always more receptive to a person's aura if we have just massaged that person. At the same time, the recipient of your massage will also be more receptive to the energies emanating from you. This brings us to the final, and possibly the most important aspect in healing: empathy between healer and recipient.

EMPATHY

When receiving professional aromatherapy treatment – especially aromatherapy massage – it is important to feel at ease with your therapist if it is to be of any worth. The same can be said of receiving intuitive aromatherapy massage from a friend. If carried out with sensitivity rather than in a stiff and mechanical way, aromatherapy massage is a potent form of hands-on healing. Of course, it is equally important for your therapist to feel at ease with you, to facilitate an exchange of energies, as it were.

Although essential oils can help the skin and the emotions, for example, without the aid of a therapist, for deep-rooted emotional and physical problems, hands-on healing is far superior if not essential for true healing to take place. However, as we have seen in Chapter 3, clinical aromatherapy (without the use of massage) can work wonders if applied in a *holistic* rather than a *symptomatic* way.

Finally, the therapist cannot take all the credit for his or her successes; the healer is merely a catalyst in the process. No one can be healed if at one level (often on an unconscious level) they do not wish to be healed, or if they cannot trust, or let go of any fears that

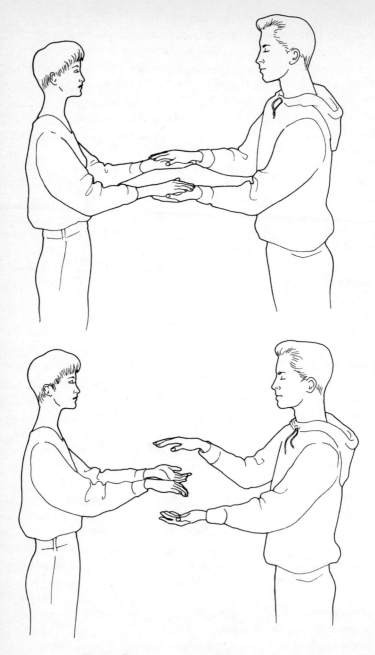

Fig. 1. Detecting auric energy

may be blocking the flow of healing energies. Every therapist/healer, orthodox or otherwise, has come across the person who just does not get better – despite doing everything 'right'.

In many cases though, the body-mind-spirit will heal itself if given the chance. By creating favourable conditions at *every* level, healing will take place quite naturally.

5

Therapeutic and Aesthetic Blending

CONCOCTING massage oils, fragrant creams and mind bending perfumes is nothing less than alchemy – your humble kitchen will never be the same again!

The big essential oil suppliers stock a bewildering array of essences. While most of these oils are suitable for aromatherapy massage, a few alas, are not (see page 126).

Essential oils are not always cheap, especially rose and neroli, but because they are highly concentrated, in use a little goes a very long way. The concentrated aroma of a neat essence can be over-powering if sniffed from the bottle, especially ylang-ylang; but once diluted, the fragrance becomes much more characteristic of the living plant – though not identical. The process of distillation tends to alter the aroma to a degree.

The essential oils listed below are the oils used in my own practice. Included in this list is some information regarding the usual method of extraction for individual oils, and some hints on aroma compatibility which you may find helpful when you come to blend essences for therapeutic as well as aesthetic purposes. I have chosen to avoid aromatic substances known as *absolutes* and *resinoids* because these are usually extracted by the employment of environmentally unfriendly solvents such as benzene.

The essences marked with an asterisk are the oils I tend to use more often. If you can afford to buy only one essence at first, choose a herbal one such as lavender or rosemary (preferably organic). These two essences are very versatile having a myriad of therapeutic properties.

44

Essential Oil	Method of Extraction	Blends well with
Basil	Steam distillation of the flowering tops	bergamot, geranium, petitgrain, coriander
˙Bergamot	Expression of oil from rind of fruit (citrus)	most essences, especially lavender, chamomile, juniper, frankincense, ylang-ylang
˙Chamomile (Roman)	Steam distillation of flowers	bergamot, rose, lavender, lemon, patchouli, neroli, petitgrain, taget
Clary-Sage (French organic)	Steam distillation of entire plant	cypress, petitgrain, juniper, citrus oils, neroli
˙Cedarwood (Virginian)	Distillation of wood	cypress, juniper, neroli, petitgrain
Coriander	Distillation of fruit (seeds)	citrus oils, neroli, cypress, ginger
˙Cypress	Distillation of leaves and cones	juniper, bergamot, sandalwood, pine needle, clary-sage
Eucalyptus	Steam distillation of leaves	lemon, lavender, pine, cypress
Fennel (sweet)	Distillation of fruit (seeds)	lemon, lavender, geranium, sandalwood
Ginger	Steam distillation of roots	citrus oils, coriander, patchouli
˙Frankincense	Distillation of the 'tears' (hardened exudations from tree)	lavender, myrrh, neroli, rose, sandalwood, citrus oils
˙Geranium (Egyptian)	Distillation of entire plant	most essences, especially citrus, neroli, juniper, petitgrain, lavender
˙Juniper (French organic)	Steam distillation of berries	citrus oils, lavender, cypress, rosemary, geranium
˙Lavender (wild, French organic)	Steam distillation of entire plant	most essences, especially chamomile, ylang-ylang, fennel, juniper, marjoram

Essential Oil	Method of Extraction	Blends well with
Lemon	Expression of oil from rind of fruit	frankincense, chamomile, ylang-ylang, bergamot, petitgrain, neroli, ginger
Marjoram (sweet)	Steam distillation of flowering tops	lavender, bergamot, rosemary
Myrrh	Distillation of hardened exudations from bush	frankincense, sandalwood, cedarwood, patchouli, coriander, ginger
Neroli	Steam or vacuum distillation of orange blossom	citrus oils, chamomile, lavender, frankincense, sandalwood, cedarwood, rose
Orange	Expression of oil from rind of fruit	frankincense, coriander, ginger
˙Patchouli	Steam distillation of the dried leaves	bergamot, geranium, lavender, myrrh, neroli, pine needle, rose, ginger
Petitgrain	Distillation of leaves from the orange tree	cheap alternative to neroli where similar aroma is required
Peppermint	Steam distillation of flowering tops and leaves	lavender, rosemary
Pine Needle	Distillation of needles and cones	cedarwood, rosemary, patchouli
Rose Otto (Bulgarian)	Steam or vacuum distillation of petals	many essences, especially sandalwood, frankincense, patchouli, clary-sage
˙Rosemary (French organic)	Distillation of leaves and flowering tops	herbal oils, cedarwood, frankincense
˙Sandalwood (Mysore)	Steam distillation of heartwood (not bark)	most essences, especially rose, ylang-lang, neroli

Essential Oil	Method of Extraction	Blends well with
Taget	Steam distillation of flowers	petitgrain, clary-sage, chamomile, citrus oils
Tea-Tree	Distillation of leaves	lemon, lavender, pine
˙Ylang-Ylang	Distillation of the flowers	most essences, especially patchouli, sandalwood, bergamot, lemon

CHOOSING AN ESSENTIAL OIL

The basic methods for using essential oils for health and skin-care are to be found in Chapter 6, but before choosing an essential oil for therapeutic or aesthetic purposes, it is important to follow the correct guidelines.

1. If you are looking for an essence (or a blend of essences) for a health problem or for skin care, consult the therapeutic cross-references or the skin care chart in this chapter.
2. When choosing an essence to help an emotional state, it is important to be guided by your aroma preference. Although certain oils are believed to be 'uplifting', 'sedative' or 'anti-depressant', it is not always as straightforward as this. The mind is much more powerful than the aroma of an essential oil. If you dislike an aroma, no matter what its 'mood-enhancing' properties may be, you are less likely to respond to its charms! Aroma preference is less important in the symptomatic treatment of basic physical problems such as athlete's foot or sprains – though some aromatherapists would disagree.
3. MOST IMPORTANT: whether you are choosing an essential oil for health or pleasure, check that the essence is safe to use; for example, if you are pregnant, avoid basil or myrrh (see page 126).

CARING FOR ESSENTIAL OILS

Essential oils evaporate readily and are easily damaged by light, extremes of temperature and prolonged exposure to oxygen in the air. Always buy essences sold in well-stoppered dark glass bottles.

In theory, most essential oils (except orange, lemon, grapefruit and lime) will keep for several years. Patchouli is unusual in that it actually improves with age, and a twenty-year-old oil will be extremely mellow and fragrant. However, the more often you open the bottle of any essential oil, the greater the chance of oxidation and thus the reduction in the oil's therapeutic properties. If stored carefully though, in a cool, dark, dry place (preferably a fridge) they will keep for at least one year (from one harvest to the next) with no problem at all.

Once diluted in vegetable oil, however, they will keep for no longer than two months, maybe three if you add a 5 per cent proportion of wheatgerm oil to the vegetable oil base. Wheatgerm oil has antioxidant properties (because of its high vitamin E content) and will help stretch marks and ageing skin. Otherwise, you could add the contents of two vitamin E capsules to every 50 ml of base oil. Finally, do check that an essential oil labelled as such is in fact 100 per cent essential oil and not one that has been diluted in almond oil (this is sometimes the case with expensive oils such as rose or neroli).

ABOUT BASE OR CARRIER OILS

Essential oils intended for aromatherapy massage need to be diluted in a natural base oil such as almond, grapeseed, peach or apricot kernel – preferably cold-pressed. Cold-pressed oils are rich in fat soluble nutrients (vitamins A, D and E) which can easily be absorbed by the skin and utilised by the body. Avoid mineral oil because it lacks the living qualities of vegetable oil and may even rob the body of some of its fat soluble nutrients.

Although aromatherapists tend to favour odourless base oils such as those mentioned above, there is no reason why you should not use a naturally fragrant oil such coconut which is lovely with rose or ylang-ylang. The jar, however, needs to be heated in a bowl of warm water before adding the essential oil because coconut oil is solid at room temperature, though it melts on contact with the skin. Lemon or bergamot blends well with sesame as a base oil; lavender and/or rosemary is good with olive oil.

MIXING MASSAGE OILS

If you intend to mix only enough oil for a single massage, use a 5 ml plastic medicine spoon (available from chemists) to measure the vegetable oil. An ordinary teaspoon will do at a pinch, though they generally hold less than 5 ml. Essential oils need to be diluted at a rate of ½ to 3 per cent, depending on the person's skin, the strength of the essential oil and the condition for which it is being applied. The lowest concentrations (½ to 2 per cent) are used for facial oils, children, and for those with sensitive skin. If your skin is sensitive, it is best to start with a ½ per cent concentration and, if this causes no irritation, increase to 1 per cent, then to 2 per cent if desired. However, a few essential oils are very strong and should never be used by anyone in concentrations above 1 to 1 ½ per cent (see page 126).

Facial Oils: For a ½ per cent concentration add *one* drop of essential oil to every *two* 5 ml teaspoonsful of base oil. For a 1 or 2 per cent concentration, add one or two drops of essential oil to each teaspoonful of base oil.

Body Oils: For a 2 or 3 per cent concentration, add two or three drops of essential oil to each teaspoonful of base oil.

For larger quantities of facial or massage oil to be stored in dark glass bottles, fill a 50 ml bottle with base oil, then add the required amount of essential oil. For a ½ per cent concentration, add 5 drops to 50 ml of base oil. For a 1 per cent concentration in the same amount of base oil, add 10 drops of essential oil; for a 2 per cent concentration, add 20 drops and for 3 per cent, add 30 drops.

Incidentally, dark glass bottles in various sizes are available from most chemists, otherwise recycle any suitable dark glass bottle with a screw cap. The capacity in mls is usually imprinted into the glass at the base of the bottle.

ABOUT BLENDING

There are no rigid rules about blending, at least as far as aromatherapy is concerned – though perfumers may disagree. It is all a matter of taste, and more importantly, a matter of how an aroma makes you feel. What does it make you think of? Is it a feeling you would like to have more often?

Of course, there is no reason why you should not use a single essential oil if you are intrigued by its aroma (rose, sandalwood and ylang-ylang are popular used singly), though aromatherapists have always felt they work better blended with other essences. Interestingly, this intuitive response has been borne out by science (see page 8).

In very simple terms, a 'well-balanced' perfume is composed of *top notes, middle notes* and *base notes*, just like music. The top notes are highly volatile; they do not last very long (coriander, citrus oils). The middle notes last a little longer (rose, neroli); and the base notes have a profound influence on the blend. They are very long-lasting, and at the same time, they 'fix' other essences. This means they slow down the volatility rate of the top and middle notes thus improving on the 'staying power' of the perfume. Sandalwood is the base note regarded by many perfumers as a good fixative because it harmonises well as a background to a wide variety of blends.

Now, you can choose to ignore all this about perfume notes if you wish – many aromatherapists do! Although it helps in making lovely perfumes if you are adventurous with a modicum of artistic flair *anyone* can concoct pleasant blends once they become confident enough to experiment. If you are totally perplexed about blending, however, remember that 'families' of essences generally blend harmoniously: herbs (basil, clary-sage, lavender, marjoram, rosemary), citrus (bergamot, lemon, orange), flowers (rose, ylang-ylang, chamomile, taget). Other compatible blends are spices with citrus (coriander and ginger with bergamot) and blends of woody essences (sandalwood with cypress). Woods and resins are a good match too: frankincense with cedarwood is a classic. But why not be much more adventurous and try blending totally unrelated essences such as frankincense with rose or lavender; neroli with clary-sage; sandalwood with lemon and ylang-ylang. Incidentally, when using very penetrating essences such as ylang-ylang, taget and especially ginger, go easy – otherwise they will overpower the blend.

Before going ahead and mixing a perfume as directed in the 'Aromatic Concoctions' section, the easiest and perhaps the most economical way to experiment is to put a few drops on a *damp* cotton wool stick. If you dislike the aroma, you have only wasted a tiny amount of essential oil. For example: try two drops of bergamot, one drop of lavender and one drop of sandalwood. If this aroma is appealing, blend into a perfume (see page 69) at the rate of 10 drops of bergamot and 5 drops each of lavender and sandalwood.

By blending different essential oils, we not only improve the aroma of a single essence, but more interestingly, we can control the mind-body effect of the oil. For instance, you may be feeling depressed and lethargic, yet love the gentle, relaxing aroma of sandalwood. However, you may benefit from a more stimulating, uplifting aroma. This could be achieved by blending the sandalwood with a little fennel, geranium or pine-needle, depending on your aroma preference (refer to the chart below).

To take another example, you may be suffering from the kind of depression that results in anxiety and insomnia as well as aching muscles (as is most common). Therefore, you will need a muscle relaxant (refer to the Therapeutic Charts in this chapter), sedative, anti-depressant blend such as chamomile and lavender. To cheer this up a little or to add an interesting note, you could add a touch of ylang-ylang, taget, bergamot or perhaps frankincense. The possibilities are, in fact, endless; there is always a blend to suit the ever-changing pattern of the mind-body.

The following chart categorises the essential oils listed at the beginning of this chapter according to their perfume 'notes'. It also includes the generally accepted mind-body or *psychosomatic* influence of each oil. However, we need to keep an open mind about this because people can respond differently to each essence.

KEY: T (Top Note), M (Middle Note), B (Base Note).

Relaxing	Balancing (stimulates or relaxes according to needs)	Stimulating
Chamomile M	Bergamot T	Basil T
Clary-Sage M	Geranium M	Coriander T
Cedarwood B		Eucalyptus T
Cypress T	Frankincense B	Fennel M
Juniper M		Ginger M
Marjoram M		Lemon T
Myrrh M		Peppermint T
Neroli M		Pine Needle M
Patchouli B		Rosemary M
Rose Otto M		Tea-Tree T
Sandalwood B		
Taget M		
Ylang-Ylang M		

Anti-Depressant	Aphrodisiac	Anaphrodisiac (*a turn-off!*)
Basil T	Coriander T	Marjoram M
Bergamot T	Ginger M	
Chamomile M	Neroli M	
Clary-Sage M	Patchouli B	
Frankincense B	Rose Otto M	
Geranium M	Sandalwood B	
Lavender M	Ylang-Ylang M	
Lemon T		*Mental Stimulant*
Neroli M		(for clarity of
Orange T		thought)
Patchouli B		Basil T
Petitgrain T		Peppermint T
Rose Otto M		Rosemary M
Sandalwood B		
Ylang-Ylang M		

Always remember that too much of *any* essence can be over stimulating, or in the opposite extreme, stupefying – so please use the oils in the correct concentrations (see page 48).

THE THERAPEUTIC CHARTS

Over the next several pages you will find a therapeutic cross-reference suggesting treatments and oils to be used for a variety of specific ailments. There is also a skin-care chart outlining remedies for skin problems. Although aromatherapy can help many ailments, it works best in the context of a holistic health regime. By this I mean we need to look to the cause of the problem, not just to the symptoms which can sometimes be the signs of a more serious underlying health problem (see Chapter 7). Above all though, aromatherapy is about the prevention of illness.

Other forms of gentle therapy such as yoga and medical herbalism have been suggested where appropriate, any of which can be used in conjunction with aromatherapy. Homoeopathy is the exception and is recommended as an alternative therapy should treatment with essential oils and herbs be only partially effective. Many homoeopaths are of the opinion that most essential oils antidote or weaken the healing effect of homoeopathic remedies – though this is very much a subject of debate. Marguerite Maury, the pioneer of holistic aromatherapy, and her husband Dr E.A. Maury, often successfully combined the two therapies.[6]

Instead of taking essences by mouth to help certain health problems (as advocated by some aromatherapists) I have suggested herb teas where appropriate. It is best for the layperson to avoid internal doses of essential oils (unless under the guidance of a well-qualified aromatherapist or herbalist) because they are very strong.

Preparing Herbal Medicines

Infusion (tea):   Put 15 g dried herbs into a warmed china or pyrex vessel. Pour over 600 ml of boiling water and allow to steep for 10–15 minutes. If you use fresh herbs, generally you will need three times as much. Seeds such as fennel should be bruised before being made into an infusion to release the essential oils from the cells.

Dosage: For general conditions, take a wineglassful three times a day every four hours.

Decoction: This is used for hard and woody plant material such as roots, rhizomes and barks. Put 15 g of dried plant material, or 45 g of fresh, broken into small pieces, into an enamel saucepan or other heatproof vessel. *Never use aluminium* as poisonous seepage will react with the plant alkaloids and its vitamin content, thus damaging the therapeutic properties. Pour over 300 ml of water and simmer with the lid on for 10 to 15 minutes.

Dosage: Same as an infusion.

Although the charts are in no way comprehensive (essential oils can help a great many more health problems) they serve as an example as well as a self-help guide to the home treatment of a number of common ailments.

THERAPEUTIC CROSS REFERENCE

The following pages show tables of Therapeutic Cross References.

Problem	Essential Oils	Method of Application	Further Suggestions
Circulation			
Cellulite	juniper, cypress, rosemary, lavender, lemon, fennel	baths, massage	See 'Anti-cellulite programme' in Chapter 5. Herb Teas: dandelion, vervain, nettle
Chilblains	lavender, lemon	massage, baths, hand/footbaths, ointment	For ointment recipe, see 'aromatic concoctions' section Broken chilblains: apply neat lavender essence
Poor circulation	juniper, cypress, ginger, lavender, orange, lemon	massage, baths	Adequate exercise, skin brushing, deep breathing exercises. Herb teas: yarrow, thyme
High blood pressure	lavender, ylang-ylang	baths, massage, skin & room perfumes with any relaxing essences	Take 2 garlic capsules daily. Seek advice from holistic therapist. Seek to reduce the stress in your life

Problem	Essential Oils	Method of Application	Further Suggestions
Constipation	rose, rosemary marjoram, fennel	baths, massage (especially over abdomen with circular strokes, clockwise direction following shape of colon)	Plenty of fresh air and exercise. Seek to reduce the stress in your life; read *The Wright Diet* (see appendix)
Women's problems Menopause (hot flushes, mood swings)	cypress, clary-sage, geranium, chamomile, fennel	baths, massage, skin and room perfumes with relaxing, uplifting essences	Deep breathing, relaxation, pollen tablets, Herb teas: black cohosh, fennel and sage (reduces hot flushes) seek professional help if symptoms are severe.
P.M.S. (pre-menstrual syndrome)	geranium, juniper, cypress, chamomile, lavender, frankincense, sandalwood, cedarwood	massage, baths, room and skin perfumes	Efamol (evening primrose oil with zinc, B6, magnesium, vitamin C). Available as a pre-menstrual pack from chemists and health food shops. Yoga, deep relaxation. Herb tea: *vitex agnus castus* (chastetree)
First-Aid Bruises	fennel, marjoram	cold compress, essential oil ointment.	For ointment recipe see 'aromatic concoctions' section

55

Problem	Essential Oils	Method of Application	Further Suggestions
Burns and scalds	lavender	apply neat to small burns, as a compress to larger burns	Cool burns immediately under cold, running water. Serious burns need urgent medical attention. Rescue Remedy (Bach Flower)
Sprains	eucalyptus, lavender, rosemary	cold compress, essential oil ointment	Apply ointment containing appropriate oils to aid healing. See 'aromatic concoctions' section
Insect stings (including wasps, bees and ants)	lavender tea-tree	apply neat	Lavender can also neutralise the poison of the black widow spider and possibly snake venom!
Wounds, cuts and grazes	most essences, especially tea-tree and lavender	apply neat essence or add 10 drops to 50 ml of water and sprinkle onto a lint dressing	To aid healing, apply an essential oil ointment; recipe in 'aromatic concoctions' section

Problem	Essential Oils	Method of Application	Further Suggestions
Mouth			
Gingivitis	tea-tree, myrrh, cypress	mouthwash	Visit your dentist! (See mouthwash recipe in 'aromatic concoctions' section)
Mouth ulcers	tea-tree, myrrh, cypress	mouthwash (as above)	Reduce the stress in your life take 1 g of vitamin C daily and a strong B-complex formula
Hair and scalp			
Dandruff	chamomile, juniper, rosemary, lavender, tea-tree, eucalyptus	scalp massage, hair and scalp oil, hair tonics	If severe (saborrheic dermatitis) which appears thick and greasy, seek dietary advice from holistic therapist. Other therapy: Homoeopathy See 'aromatic concoctions' section
Headlice	lavender, rosemary, tea-tree, eucalyptus	hair oil	See 'aromatic concoctions' section

Problem	Essential Oils	Method of Application	Further Suggestions
Muscles and joints Over-worked, aching muscles	lavender, eucalyptus, rosemary, juniper, cypress, marjoram, chamomile, pine-needle,	baths, massage, warm compress	Regular massage helps prevent muscle pain and the development of arthritis, especially if you do a lot of sport and are forced to give up suddenly
Arthritis and rheumatism	chamomile, cypress, ginger, marjoram, rosemary, lemon eucalyptus, juniper, coriander lavender	baths, massage, ointment, foot/hand baths where appropriate (alternate *hot* and *cold*, finishing with *cold* to prevent enervation of the skin over inflamed areas)	Diet is very important. It would be advisable to seek professional advice or read *The Wright Diet* In arthritis, never massage *inflamed* joints – it is usually too painful to do so, anyway! Sunshine, swimming, air and salt water helps. **Other therapies:** acupuncture, naturopathy, osteopathy, chiropractic, herbalism, homoeopathy, yoga. Herbal preparation: devil's claw (available in tablet form). See 'aromatic concoctions' for ointment recipe

Problem	Essential Oils	Method of Application	Further Suggestions
Respiratory Colds, 'flu, sinusitis, coughs	juniper eucalyptus, tea-tree, peppermint, pine-needle, marjoram, lavender, lemon, garlic (capsules), cloves, cinnamon (room fumigant only)	baths, steam inhalations, massage oil for chest, room fumigation with blend of lavender, eucalyptus and cloves.	1) For colds and 'flu: honey, lemon and grated ginger root (to taste) in hot water. Drink three times daily. 2) As a preventative remedy for respiratory ailments, take 2 garlic capsules and 2 × 500 mg vitamin C daily. 3) For coughs: 2 drops of eucalyptus, lavender or juniper in a teacupful of water to be used as a gargle 3 times daily. For sinusitis: facial massage helps
Catarrh	lavender, myrrh sandalwood, chamomile, eucalyptus, rosemary, frankincense	baths, massage, steam inhalations	For chronic catarrh, seek the aid of a holistic therapist. As a preventative, 2–3 garlic capsules daily and 2 × 500 mg of vitamin C; cut down on dairy products. Herb teas: yarrow, lemon balm, ginger (decoction), peppermint

Problem	Essential Oils	Method of Application	Further Suggestions
Skin Acne	Local: chamomile, juniper, lavender, sandalwood eucalyptus, tea-tree, rosemary. General: (baths and massage) geranium, neroli, rose, lemon, bergamot	facial oils and/or skin tonics, steam inhalations, body massage, baths	Holistic treatment is necessary Seek guidance of a qualified aromatherapist if self-help is unsuccessful. Other therapies: herbalism naturopathy, homoeopathy Read *The Wright Diet*. Herb teas: dandelion, horsetail, fenugreek, burdock, poke root (decoction), nettle. See 'aromatic concoctions' section for skin-tonic recipe
Athlete's foot	tea-tree, lavender, lemon	neat essence applied to affected parts or use an essential oil ointment, footbaths	Expose feet to sunshine and fresh air as often as possible. For ointment recipe, see 'aromatic concoctions' section
Scabies	peppermint, lavender, rosemary, tea-tree	ointment, baths	Apply ointment 3 times daily and take 3–6 garlic capsules daily until problem has cleared. For ointment recipe, see 'aromatic concoctions' section

Problem	Essential Oils	Method of Application	Further Suggestions
Ringworm	tea-tree, geranium	ointment	Apply ointment 3 times daily. See 'aromatic concoctions' for ointment recipe
Eczema	chamomile, lavender Weeping eczema: juniper	baths, general massage (not over affected areas), beeswax ointment containing a low concentration of essential oils	Holistic treatment is necessary. Seek professional help. Read *The Wright Diet*. Other therapies: herbalism, yoga, Bach Flower Remedies, allergy testing, homoeopathy. Herb teas: chamomile, red clover, nettle, marigold. See 'aromatic concoctions' section for ointment recipe
Stress Anxiety	bergamot, chamomile, cypress, geranium, frankincense, sandalwood, juniper, marjoram, patchouli, rose, clary-sage, ylang-ylang, taget	baths, massage, skin and room perfumes	*Read Chapter 7* Long-term anxiety or depression needs the help of a holistic therapist. Other therapies: Bach Flower Remedies, Psychotherapy, counselling, yoga

Problem	Essential Oils	Method of Application	Further Suggestions
Depression	bergamot, chamomile, lemon, orange, coriander, geranium, lavender, neroli, petitgrain, sandalwood, clary-sage, patchouli, rose, ylang-ylang, taget	As above	As above
Insomnia	all the essences listed for anxiety, especially chamomile and lavender	As above	As above
Headache	chamomile, lavender, rose, rosemary, marjoram, peppermint	head, face and neck massage. Sniff a bottle of peppermint essence	There are many possible causes of headache too numerous to mention here. Continual, migraine-type headaches should be investigated by a medical practitioner. Herb teas: peppermint, chamomile, skullcap, rosemary

SKIN-CARE CHART

Dry Skin	Oily Skin/Acne	Ageing Skin
Rose	Rosemary	Frankincense
Chamomile	Lavender	Myrrh
Sandalwood	Cypress	Rose
Lavender	Juniper	Sandalwood
Neroli	Lemon	Neroli
	Geranium	
	Frankincense	
	Tea-tree	

Thread Veins	Combination Skin	Normal Skin
Rose	Geranium	Lavender
Chamomile	Lavender	Rose
Lemon	Rose	Chamomile
Cypress	Chamomile	Neroli
		Geranium
		Frankincense

Puffy Skin (water-logged)	Sensitive Skin	Dehydrated Skin (especially after tanning)
Juniper	Try ½ per cent	Lavender
Cypress	concentrations of	Geranium
Geranium	Lavender	Chamomile
Lavender	Rose	Rose
Lemon	Chamomile	
	(see also 'allergies' page 126)	

AROMATIC CONCOCTIONS

The following recipes are a selection of my own aromatic concoctions; no doubt you will invent many more!

Massage Oil for Cellulite

50 ml of grapeseed oil (or any other vegetable oil), 10 drops of juniper, 10 drops of lavender, 5–10 drops of lemon.

Method: Funnel the grapeseed oil into a dark glass bottle, add the essential oils and shake well. This oil also makes a very good blend for aching muscles and joints.

Treatment for Head Lice

75ml (3 fl oz) vegetable oil, 25 drops of tea-tree or eucalyptus, 25 drops of lavender, 25 drops of rosemary. Mix as for previous recipe.

How to use: Apply to wet hair (otherwise it will be difficult to shampoo out the oil) by massaging well into the scalp to reach the hair roots. Pay particular attention to the areas around the ears and nape of the neck where the lice breed. Leave on for about an hour, then shampoo thoroughly. Remove the eggs (nits) with a regulation fine-toothed comb. Repeat twice at three-day intervals.

Pre-Wash Hair Oil for Dry or Damaged Hair

50 ml olive oil, 10 drops of sandalwood, 10 drops of lavender, 5 drops of geranium. Mix as for previous recipes.

How to use: Apply to wet hair; leave on for 15–30 minutes before shampooing out. Use as a weekly conditioning treatment.

Hair Oil for Dandruff

50 ml of olive oil, 10 drops of rosemary, 10 drops of lavender, 5 drops of tea-tree or juniper. Mix as for previous recipes.

How to use: Apply to wet hair; massage into the scalp and leave on for 15–30 minutes. Shampoo thoroughly. Use as a weekly treatment. If your hair is oily, use an anti-dandruff hair tonic instead (see page 65).

HAIR TONICS

These are massaged into the scalp several times a week. There is no need to wet your hair first. If used regularly, they will improve the condition of your hair and scalp. Cider vinegar is included in all the recipes to restore the acid/alkali balance of the scalp. All hair tonics need to be shaken before use to disperse the essences which are only partially soluble in water.

Anti-Dandruff Tonic

300 ml distilled water or orange flower water or rosewater or 50/50 distilled water and witch hazel, 3 teaspoonsful of cider vinegar, 6 drops of lavender, 6 drops of rosemary, 3 drops of juniper or tea-tree.

Method: Funnel the distilled water and cider vinegar into a dark glass bottle, add the essences and shake well.

Tonic for Thinning Hair

While this tonic may not be a cure for male-pattern baldness, if used regularly, following the scalp massage instructions in Chapter 6, it may halt the process. You need 300 ml rosewater, 3 teaspoonsful of cider vinegar, 7 drops of rosemary, 5 drops sandalwood. Mix as for previous recipe.

SKIN TONICS

As for hair tonics, you will need to shake well before use to disperse the essential oils.

Skin Tonic Base

300 ml of rosewater or orange flower water or distilled water. For very oily skin or acne, you could use a more astringent base such as witch hazel. This could be made slightly less astringent by mixing it 50/50 with a flower water or distilled water. To the flower water

or distilled water, add 2 teaspoonsful of cider vinegar, then add 2 drops of the appropriate essential oil for your skin-type (refer to the skin-care chart on page 63). Use as suggested in the skin-care section in Chapter 6.

MOUTHWASH

This is a healing, antiseptic mixture to strengthen the gums. It will also help to heal mouth ulcers and prevent the onset of gingivitis. Use 30 ml tincture of myrrh (available from herbalists), 10 drops of peppermint or fennel, 15 drops of tea-tree.

How to use: 6–8 drops in a small teacupful of warm water two or three times a day.

FACE-PACKS

Most skin (except the very sensitive) will benefit from an application of live, full-fat natural yogurt, even without the addition of essential oils (see page 77). The following recipe will cleanse, brighten and tighten the skin and is suitable for 'normal', combination and ageing complexions.

Ingredients: 3 teaspoonsful of live, full-fat yogurt, 1 teaspoonful of cold-pressed almond, olive or hazelnut oil, 1 drop of essential oil for your skin-type (see skin-care chart, page 63). About ½ to 1 teaspoonful of fine oatmeal to bind.

Method: Mix the essential oil into the base oil and stir in the other ingredients to form a paste.

How to use: Apply a thin layer to the face and neck and leave on for 10–15 minutes. Rinse off with cool water.

For Dry Skin

¼ ripe avocado, ½ teaspoonful of avodado or wheatgerm oil, 1 drop of chamomile or rose, about ½ a teaspoonful of fine oatmeal to bind.

Method: Mix the essential oil with the base oil. Mash the avocado to a pulp and stir in the oils. Mix in a little oatmeal to bind.

How to use: As for previous recipe, but rinse off with tepid water.

For Oily Skin and Acne

1 teaspoonful of live, natural yoghurt, 1 teaspoonful of brewer's yeast powder, ½ teaspoon of warm water (more if necessary), ½ teaspoon of cold-pressed almond oil, 1 drop of lavender, juniper or lemon.

Method: Mix the essential oil into the almond oil and stir into the other ingredients to form a paste.

How to use: Preferably after a bath or facial sauna (congested skin does not readily absorb substances unless warm and moist). Apply to face and neck, leave on for 10–15 minutes and rinse off with cool water.

MAKING SKIN CREAMS AND OINTMENTS

Home-made skin creams are richer and heavier than the super-light 'mousse' creations available at the cosmetics counter, but they are extremely effective and economical. The following recipe makes a fairly soft cream which will harden slightly if kept in the fridge (to halt the formation of mould), but nevertheless melts on contact with the skin. You will find a tiny amount will go a long way. Use it as a hand-cream or face-cream for drier skin.

You can experiment with other vegetable oils in the blend (hazelnut, apricot kernal) as long as they add up to 120 ml in all. A proportion of wheatgerm oil added to the formula (20 ml) will increase the shelf-life and enhance its healing properties. All home-made creams and ointments will keep for several months if stored in a cool dark place. Yellow beeswax (used in the cream and ointment recipe) is more natural than white beeswax. This is obtainable from herbal suppliers.

Basic Skin Cream

15 g yellow beeswax
120 ml almond oil
30 ml distilled water or rosewater or orangeflower water
4–6 drops of essential oil (see skin-care chart, page 63)

1. Melt the beeswax with the oil in the top of an enamel double boiler or heat-proof basin over a pan of simmering water.
2. Meanwhile, heat the distilled water in another basin over a pan of simmering water until it has warmed. There is no need to be too precise about temperature, but blood heat is about right.
3. Begin to add the warm distilled water, drop by drop at first, to the oil and wax, beating with a rotary whisk, balloon whisk or an electric food mixer *set at the lowest speed.*
4. After you have mixed about two teaspoonsful of the water into the oil and wax, remove from the heat and continue adding the water a little at a time until you have incorporated it all.
5. As soon as the mixture begins to set, stir in the essences.
6. Divide the mixture into little sterilized glass pots and cover tightly.

Basic Ointment (Pomade)

15 g yellow beeswax
60 ml almond oil
10–15 drops of essential oil (refer to Therapeutic Cross-Reference, page 54)

Heat the beeswax and almond oil in a double enamel boiler or in a heatproof dish over a pan of simmering water. Stir well, remove from the heat and when cool, add the essential oils. Pour into a sterilized glass pot and cover tightly.

Important: For infectious skin problems such as athlete's foot, scabies and ringworm you will need to double the quantity of essential oils, or apply neat lavender or tea-tree oil.

AROMATIC WATERS AND PERFUMES

Here you can become wild and creative, concocting exotic, relaxing or simply herbal blends as your moods dictate.

The aromatic waters can be used in the same way as commercial products – splashed on after a bath or shower. Natural perfumes need to be diluted in a bland vegetable oil – soya, corn or grapeseed – or in jojoba wax. The latter is best, though expensive, because unlike vegetable oil, it does not go off. Commercial perfumes and aromatic waters are diluted in ethyl alcohol which is not generally available (at least in Britain) without a perfumer's licence.

How to Make an Aromatic Water

In 100 ml of orange flower water, rosewater or distilled water, add up to 100 drops of essential oil. Shake well each time before use. Here are a few of my own concoctions to give you some ideas:

Mandelay: (an oriental-type aroma, very cheering and seductive). To the flower water or distilled water base, add 16 drops ylang-ylang, 40 drops bergamot, 30 drops patchouli, 10 drops coriander *or* ginger.

Moments: (a softly sensual, flowery/woody aroma). To the fluid base, add 55 drops sandalwood, 15 drops cedarwood, 15 drops rose, 4 drops taget, 15 drops ylang-ylang.

Skin Perfumes

Use up to 25 drops of essential oil to a 10 ml base of jojoba wax or vegetable oil.

Mock Jasmine: (this resembles the costly jasmine absolute). 15 drops of patchouli, 6 drops ylang-ylang.

Pharaoh: (rather heavy and sedate). 10 drops frankincense, 4 drops myrrh, 6 drops cedarwood, 5 drops rose.

Cottage garden: 10 drops lavender, 6 drops rose, 4 drops clary-sage, 1 or 2 drops taget.

Three Therapeutic But Nice Perfumes

1. For when you feel tense with worrying thoughts constantly invading your sleep: 10 drops bergamot, 5 drops clary-sage, 3

drops ylang-ylang. Occasionally, I add 3 drops of cedarwood to this blend which brings it down a little.

2. When you need comforting and uplifting: 10 drops sandalwood, 6 drops bergamot, 4 drops neroli.
3. For when you feel 'ungrounded', especially after a bout of flu when you may be feeling light-headed and distant: 15 drops patchouli, 5 drops ginger. I prefer this blend with about 5 drops of bergamot or lemon added to brighten the aroma.

PERFUMING ROOMS

Follow the basic suggestions for perfuming rooms as outlined on page 105. Any of the perfume blends suggested earlier can also be used to subtly influence the mood of the occupants within a room. Here are a few more ideas: to jolly up a winter's party, try a mixture of cinnamon bark, cloves and orange. Lavender, clary-sage and chamomile will aid restful sleep. For meditation, yoga or for a philosophical discussion, try a blend of frankincense, myrrh and cedarwood. A children's party will go down well with a background fragrance of bergamot, orange or lemon, and perhaps a touch of geranium.

Finally, if you are trying to sell your house, but without much success, aromatherapy may be the answer. Next time a prospective buyer comes to view, make sure the kitchen is scented with the soft fragrance of vanilla (the cooking kind). Put a few drops of natural vanilla essence into a pan of water and place in a low oven. There is nothing more seductive than vanilla which evokes in most people cosy feelings of home-baked cakes, warmth and security. Your house will be sold in no time at all!

6

The Techniques of Aromatherapy

ESSENTIAL OILS can be used in a variety of ways to promote health and vitality. They can be used in skin-care, made into massage oils, added to the bath, used in steam inhalations for colds and 'flu, blended into mood-enhancing perfumes and in other ways to enhance our daily lives. Let us start with the care of the skin.

CARING FOR THE SKIN

Caring for your skin needs to go deeper than superficial 'beauty care' confined to the face. Nor need it be an exclusively female activity, as many people would have us believe. In fact, a healthy skin is a reflection of good health in general; the skin is an accurate barometer of emotional and physical harmony and indeed, disharmony. Therefore, no amount of external treatment with the finest plant oils will help much if your diet, life-style and emotions are out of balance. First treat your skin from this perspective (see Chapter 7) and the oils will work more efficiently, adding much more than just the polish!

If, however, you suffer from a skin complaint such as eczema, psoriasis or acne, you may need to seek further advice (an aroma-therapist, herbalist or nutritionist) who will devise for you a personalised healing programme. We are all different; what may work for one individual will not necessarily work as well for another.

In simple terms, skin is far more than a superficial covering for the body; it is a living, breathing organism. It has a two-way job, that of protecting the rest of the body from infection and dirt, and that of eliminating toxins. In fact, the skin is the body's largest eliminating organ weighing about 3 kilograms, and far from being delicate, it is dynamically hard-working. If the body is healthy, cell growth and reproduction go on unceasingly.

Skin is affected by many factors including genetics, age, environment and attention – or lack of it. Even if you are one of the lucky few, blessed with a fine trouble-free skin, the use of essential oils along with the techniques outlined in this chapter will not only help to preserve its suppleness for as long as possible, but will improve your health in general.

DRY SKIN BRUSHING

The benefits of this old and well-proven European Nature Cure technique are truly staggering. Not only does it help the condition of the skin itself by removing the build-up of dead skin cells on the surface, it stimulates lymphatic drainage and the elimination of as much as one-third of body wastes. According to natural healing principles, these toxins can lead to disease if they are allowed to accumulate in the body. Complaints such as arthritis, cellulite, high-blood pressure and even depression have been linked to poor lymphatic drainage.

The lymphatic system is concerned with our immune defences (the production of antibodies against infection) and with the elimination of toxic wastes through the skin, lungs, kidneys and colon. Unlike the circulatory system, in which the circulation of the blood is controlled by the pumping of the heart, the lymph is usually kept moving by the normal contraction and relaxation of the muscles during physical activity. If you lead a sedentary life (especially if you are wheel-chair bound), or you are elderly – or simply lazy! – skin brushing is a blessing. It cannot totally replace exercise, but it is in fact the same in body stimulation terms as a good massage or twenty minutes of jogging!

In aromatherapy, skin brushing is more commonly used to combat cellulite; and combined with lymphatic drainage massage, essential oils and a detoxifying diet, it is very effective (see page 101). Furthermore, as many other natural therapists have discovered, it can be used as an all-round health aid. British herbalists Kitty Campion and Jill Davies, along with American writer and health expert Leslie Kenton, have been extolling the virtues of dry skin-brushing for years.

HOW TO DO IT

You will need a purpose designed vegetable bristle brush (nylon or animal bristle is either too soft or too rough) with a long, but detachable handle so that you can reach your back. These are available from many good health-food shops or from some chemists. It must always be kept dry but washed in warm soapy water every two weeks. The body needs to be brushed once a day for a few minutes before your morning bath or shower (twice if you have cellulite). It is a good idea to take a week's break every month as skin brushing, like many natural detoxification techniques, is more effective if the body does not become too accustomed to it.

Avoiding the face, which is too sensitive for this treatment, make bold sweeping movements over each part of the body as in Fig. 2. Be GENTLE; brush too vigorously, especially if you are new to body brushing, and you will scratch your skin. Begin with your feet, including the soles, and work up the legs, front and back, over the buttocks and up to the middle-back. That is, always work towards the heart and bring toxins towards the colon. Then brush your hands, up the arms, front and back, across the shoulders, down the chest (avoiding the nipples if you are a woman) and then down the back of the neck to the upper back. Finally, brush the abdomen (avoiding the genitals) using a *clockwise* circular motion following the shape of the colon.

Skin brushing need take no longer than five minutes each time and can be done while you run the bath. After the bath or shower, apply your favourite aromatherapy massage oil to nourish your skin – or if appropriate, an anti-cellulite oil.

Important: Skin brushing is safe for everybody, except for those suffering from skin disorders such as eczema or psoriasis or if there is infected or broken skin. You can brush where the skin is healthy, but avoid any areas where you have bad varicose veins.

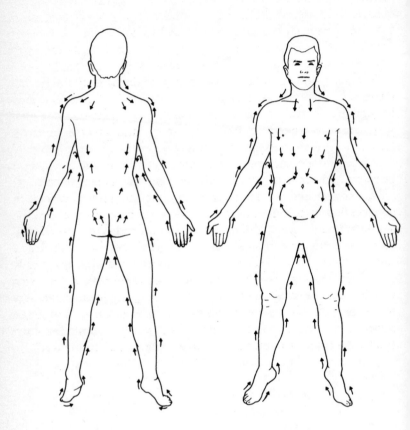

Fig. 2. Dry Skin Brushing
(Avoid the face, nipples and genitals)

THE FACE

Wash your face twice daily with a mild pH balanced soap or cleansing bar which helps to balance the skin's acid mantle. The mantle is a mixture of sebum (oil) and fluid supporting a microflora of bacteria (the skin's defence against infection). It has a pH value of 5.5 which means it is slightly acid. Ordinary soaps and cheap facial preparations are alkaline and in some people can lead to dry, flaky skin.

After washing, particularly if your skin is oily, apply a mild astringent such as rosewater (or one of the skin tonics suggested in Chapter 5). Rosewater also makes a good aftershave for men with sensitive skin. Skin tonics make the skin feel fresh and help to remove residues of soap or cleanser.

While the skin is still damp, apply a moisturiser made from beeswax and plant oils (page 68) or a good commercial product. However, avoid skin care preparations containing humectants such as glycerin, glycol, sodium pyrrolidone, propylene or carboxylic acid. Although they feel and look good on the skin at the time, by attracting water from the air, they also tend to attract water from within the outer layers of the skin too. This can easily evaporate leaving the skin taut and parchment-like. The skin can become 'hooked' on these moisturisers, craving regular fixes to feel comfortable. As most commercial moisturisers contain these substances, at least half of the female population in western society (and some of its progressive men) must be moisturiser 'junkies'!

Exfoliation

Exfoliation will improve the texture of the skin, particularly if you are over thirty. This will remove the dead skin cells on the surface of the skin which tend to block the pores causing pigmentation and a dull appearance. Younger skins tend to shed dead skin cells without help, but as we age, the reproduction processes under the skin slow down. New skin cells are formed more slowly and worn-out cells, which are pushed to the surface, tend to stay around in patches.

How to do it: Moisten a handful of medium ground oatmeal (cornmeal if your skin is dry) and use as a gentle scrub. Rub into all parts of your face and throat. Be especially attentive around the nostrils. Rinse off with warm to cool water. If you are a man and you shave, there is no need to bother with the oatmeal scrub because shaving amounts to the same thing.

Occasional Skin Treatments

Face-packs and facial saunas are good for city skins or for those times when you feel your skin needs a pick-me-up (during the winter perhaps) or to quell an eruption of spots. Skin eruptions are common to many of us during times of stress and in women during the pre-menstrual phase.

The Facial Sauna

A facial sauna is a deep cleaning treatment which is good for all skin-types, but especially for blemished and congested skin. Saunas must be avoided at all costs however if your skin is prone to thread veins. The intense heat will dilate the blood vessels lying under the skin's surface, thus exacerbating the problem. They should also be avoided if you suffer from asthma; concentrated steam may trigger an attack.

Shake one or two drops of an essence suitable for your skin-type (see page 63) into a bowl containing ½ litre of steaming water. Now cover your whole head with a towel and put it over the steaming bowl so the towel forms a 'tent' to catch the steam. Stay there for up to five minutes. Finish this treatment by splashing your face with cool water to remove wastes accumulated on the surface of the skin. You can follow this treatment with a face-pack, or wait half an hour for your skin to settle down and apply your usual moisturiser. A word of warning about facial saunas. American studies on skin health have indicated that the over-use of steam treatments (more than twice a week over many months) can cause 'jungle acne' – a disorder brought about by the presence of excess moisture in the skin. If used sensibly though, once a week perhaps, your skin will certainly benefit. It will begin to look and feel revitalised and dewy.

Face-Packs

A weekly face-pack, or mask as they are often called, can be applied to the face and neck after ordinary cleansing, or better still, after an aromatic bath or facial steam while the skin is still moist and warm and therefore, more receptive to whatever you put on it.

Face packs are designed to balance skin secretions, to stimulate the circulation and to moisturise and tighten the skin. One of the most beneficial substances to use as a face pack is yogurt (live, natural yogurt, full-fat if possible); beneficial, that is, if you are not allergic to dairy products. Fresh, live yogurt, without additives, can help all skin-types, particularly excessively dry or oily skin. The lactic acid of yogurt (due to its fermentation) is similar to that of the skin acid mantle, and appears to exert a balancing action on the secretion of skin fluids.

You will need about a teaspoonful of yogurt which you then apply to face and neck and leave on for ten to fifteen minutes. Rinse off with warm to cool water. You will see and feel the difference almost immediately. (See also the face-pack recipes in Chapter 5).

Facial Oils

The most effective way to use essential oils for skin-care is known in France as a cure. Essences are used as a periodic treatment; either once a week or daily for two weeks with a three to four week interval before resuming again. This prevents the skin from becoming too accustomed to the essences and failing to respond positively to them. You may have experienced something similar with shampoo: use the same one for too long and the remarkable results you may have seen at first begin to diminish after a few washes.

Returning to facial oils, you will find a skin-care chart and instructions for making these in Chapter 5. Do remember though not to exceed the recommended ½–1 per cent dilutions (at least initially) because too high a concentration of essential oil (especially strong ones such as chamomile or geranium) may irritate the more sensitive skin of the face (see also allergies on page 126). Body oils can generally be used in higher concentrations of around 3 per cent.

There are four ways of applying the oils for skin treatments:

1. Apply a fine film just after a bath or shower when your skin is still warm and moist. Do not wipe off any excess until after twenty minutes – it can take this long for the oils to be absorbed.
2. Apply half an hour after a face-pack or facial sauna. The skin needs time to settle down after these treatments in order to absorb the essential oils more efficiently.
3. Apply shortly before going for a walk in the open air (preferably the park or unpolluted country air). The combination of oxygen and essential oil is a superb skin rejuvenator.

If you opt for the once a week regime, apply the oils three times a day if possible, otherwise once a day is enough.

Instead of using a facial oil you might prefer to 'doctor' an unperfumed face cream or lotion (preferably a 'natural' product) with the appropriate oils for your skin type. Stir in 2 or 3 drops of essential oil to every 50 grams of cream or 1 or 2 drops to every 25 ml of lotion and shake well.

From my own experience, essences used in baths and general massage will help the complexion whether or not they are applied directly to the face. This is because they reach the bloodstream via the lungs and skin and work systemically, influencing the body as a whole. Very congested skin cannot absorb essential oils efficiently anyway, but when used in the bath and in general body massage they will be more easily absorbed through the softer skin of the abdomen, innersides of the thighs and upper arms.

AROMATHERAPY MASSAGE

There is no denying that a good aromatherapy massage is a truly divine experience; and giving massage can be enjoyable too. You can of course, massage the oils into your own skin and derive benefit from them, but the most pleasurable and certainly the most relaxing way is to receive massage from someone else – preferably a qualified massage therapist – though a friend with 'good hands' is more than adequate.

Some very basic massage strokes are outlined here, but they are meant only as a guide to enable you to begin to develop your own intuitive style. To learn massage from a book (even from a very much more detailed book than this) is not easy. If you intend to take it seriously, you will eventually feel the need to attend a weekend workshop or you may even wish to embark on an extended study course. Having said this, many people are superb intuitive massage therapists, and no amount of formal training will improve upon their special 'touch'.

One good reason for studying with a massage school is that you will be taught anatomy and physiology as well as useful techniques for alleviating pain, dealing with injuries, understanding why pain may be occurring in a particular area and even more importantly, when to leave well alone.

When not to Massage

Massage is contra-indicated in the following conditions: fever, inflammation (of skin or joints), skin rashes or eruptions, swellings, bruises, sprains, torn muscles and ligaments, broken bones, burns and varicose veins – in short, if it hurts, abandon the movement and move on to another area of the body. It is also generally believed that people with cancer should not be massaged because cancer cells may start to spread to the rest of the body via the lymphatic system. However, recent evidence does not appear to bear this out. Very gentle aromatherapy massage is being used in several British hospitals to help uplift the spirits of cancer patients.

The Effects of Massage

The moment you place your hands on another person's body, you begin to treat both mind and body simultaneously. The nerves awaken immediately. They relay messages to the brain which then sends out 'reaction' instructions throughout the body.

On the physical level, massage aids the elimination of toxic wastes (often the cause of muscle aches and pains) by stimulating blood circulation and lymphatic drainage. This increases oxygen to the painful areas and at the same time removes the stagnant toxic wastes such as lactic and carbonic acids which build up in the muscle fibres.

As mind and body are interrelated, the emotional effects of skilled, but *sensitive* aromatherapy massage can be profound. It can sometimes engender a state similar to that experienced by meditators.

Once the art of massage becomes second nature, you may begin to discover 'energy blocks' which usually manifest as cold areas in the body – perhaps the lower back or the abdomen. These cold areas are often the seat of deep-rooted emotions. As the tense muscles begin to relax, sometimes pent-up emotions are also freed. Some people find uncontrollable tears welling up, yet they may feel wonderfully relaxed and calm after the massage. Others may experience a light-headed sensation as if they have had a few glasses of wine; a few fall into a deep sleep!

Such responses, even the tears, are positive and beneficial for one's long-term health. It is a well-documented fact that cancer, for example, is more prevalent in those with a predisposition to depression and a tendency to bottle-up their emotions just to please others.

Nothing really beneficial can come about, however, unless there is an empathy between giver and receiver. If you are *giving* massage, you need to develop the ability to tune-in, as it were, to the needs of your partner, allowing your hands to move intuitively to any tender spots in his or her body and to soothe away the pain. Although this is largely an innate ability, particularly well developed in a few people, we can all develop sensitivity in general (which will help our massage skills) by such means as meditation, deep relaxation and nature attunements (see Chapter 7).

If you are *receiving* massage you need to learn how to accept massage graciously; that is, by trusting your partner and 'opening' to the experience. This cannot be achieved if you constantly chatter and move about. Instead, close your eyes, take a few deep breaths, then breathe out as a sigh and relax into the experience. Then, focus your attention on your partner's touch, enjoy the sensation; allow your body to go heavy and limp. Do not try to help by lifting your head for instance; when your head needs to be turned to one side in order to massage a part of your neck, let the turning be done for you. Of course, there are one or two exceptions to the no talking or moving yourself 'rule': do speak up if something your partner is doing is hurting, or if you feel cold or uncomfortable in any way. Also, when lying on your front, turn your head from one side to the other if your neck feels stiff.

Setting the Scene

A calm, comfortable setting will enhance the experience of aromatherapy massage. Work in natural daylight if possible or under a soft lamp or candelight. Harsh overhead lighting will only serve to remind you both of an operating theatre or a visit to the dentist! Aromatherapy massage is a gentle healing art, not a cold and unfeeling procedure.

The room should be very warm and draught-free; chilled muscles contract, causing a release of adrenalin – something you are trying to soothe away in the first place.

If you must play background music, keep the volume very low – your partner's senses will be especially acute – and stick to 'New Age' music which has been composed for meditation and deep relaxation. These tapes are available from the address in the appendix. As a final touch, you might like to place a vase of fresh flowers in the room; this will greatly enhance the atmosphere.

The Massage Surface

The most comfortable surface on which to work is a purpose built massage couch. However, you may have to work at floor level, but please do not be tempted to give massage on a bed. Not only will you have to bend too much (putting an enormous strain on your back), the mattress will absorb all the necessary pressure intended for your partner's body. A sleeping bag, strip of foam rubber, thick blankets, a soft rug or duvet on the floor will provide padding under your partner. Cover this with a sheet or towel. A second sheet or thick towel will be needed to cover areas of the body you are not working on, thus preventing your partner from becoming chilled. When giving massage on the floor, kneel beside your partner (preferably on a carpeted floor to cushion your knees). Do not attempt to give massage at floor level when standing and bending at the waist; this is even more harmful to your back than using a bed.

The Massage Oil

When choosing a massage oil, you can, if you like, try to match your partner's needs by referring to the therapeutic charts and other information in Chapter 5. Your partner may need an oil such as rosemary for stiff muscles for instance, or a relaxing oil such as ylang-ylang. However, you may feel more inclined towards intuitive aromatherapy whereby the person is allowed to choose their own oil or blend of oils according to those they like best. Remember, we are often drawn to the essential oil we may actually need at the time. In any case, the more pleasing the aroma, the more likely we will relax into the experience of aromatherapy massage – and it is this ability to let go which is the key to the art of true healing.

Giving Massage

It would be impossible to describe full-body massage in this little book, so we will concentrate on the most important areas in aromatherapy massage, the back, head, face and neck. We will also look at a simple form of self-massage to help banish cellulite.

The Back

The back may be regarded as the gateway to the whole person – body, mind and psyche. The body's main nerves branch out from either side of the spine and supply all the internal organs: By relaxing the back muscles tension and stress levels in mind and body will be reduced. This leads to improved health and a sense of well-being.

Position your partner on his or her front, head to one side, arms relaxed at the sides or loosely bent with the hands at shoulder level. *Some people feel more comfortable with a rolled up towel or cushion under the chest and ankles.* Kneel down to one side of your partner (or stand if you are using a massage couch). *Before oiling your hands*, very gently place one hand on the crown of the head and the other at the base of the spine. Hold them there for about half a minute; then move to the feet. Hold a foot in each hand quite *firmly* (some people have tickly feet!) with your palms against the soles. This is known as *connecting*. It feels very reassuring to the person and at the same time it allows them to become accustomed to your touch. It also has a very calming effect.

1. Pour some oil into a small dish (do not pour oil onto your partner's body, it can be quite a shock), oil your hands, then rub them together to warm the oil. Place your hands at the base of the back, on either side of the spine with your fingers

relaxed, pointing towards the head. You should never apply pressure to the spine itself, but the strong muscles either side can take firm pressure. Now slide your hands up the back; move your body from the centre until you reach the neck. Slide your hands firmly across the shoulders then glide them down. As you reach the waist, pull it up gently and return smoothly to the starting point (see Fig. 3).

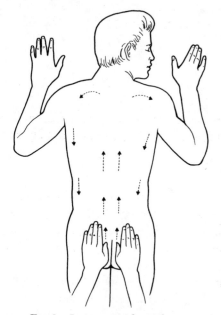

Fig. 3. Long smooth strokes

It is important to use the whole of your hands; allow them to mould the contours of your partner's body as if you were sculpting clay. Repeat these long, firm strokes several times until the whole of the back is well oiled, but not too slippery. You will find that two to four teaspoonfuls of oil will be enough for the average back. People with *very* dry skin may need a little more.

2. Now move your hands to the sides of the body and, starting from the hips (or buttocks), begin to knead. Using each hand alternately, take hold of the flesh with the whole palm of your hand and fingers, pull away from the bone and squeeze as if you were kneading dough. Keep the whole hand in contact

with your partner's body. Work up the sides of the torso and across the tops of the arms and shoulders. When you come to smaller areas (around the shoulder blades for instance) change to thumbs and two middle fingers, but do not pinch the flesh. Move to the other side of the body and repeat (see Fig. 4).

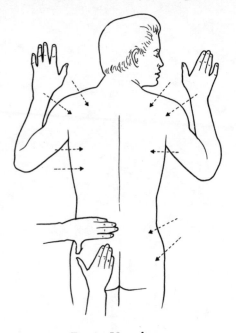

Fig.4. Kneading

3. Starting at the base of the spine, make small circular movements into the muscles either side of the spine with your thumbs until you reach the neck. With your thumbs on the upper back, continue the circular movements. Do not press on the spine or the shoulder blade itself. Work on the muscles just above the shoulder blades and those lying between them and the spine (see Fig. 5).
4. Return to the long stroke with which you began in Step 1. Repeat three times.
5. The next stroke is called pulling, and is done along the sides of the body. Move to one side of your partner's back. With your fingers pointing downwards, gently pull each hand alternately straight up from the floor or table. Start at the hip and work

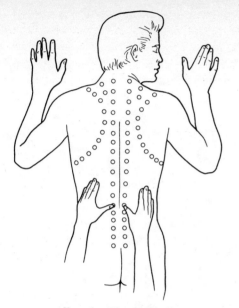

Fig. 5. Thumb circles

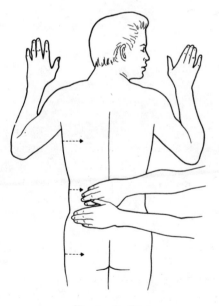

Fig. 6. Pulling

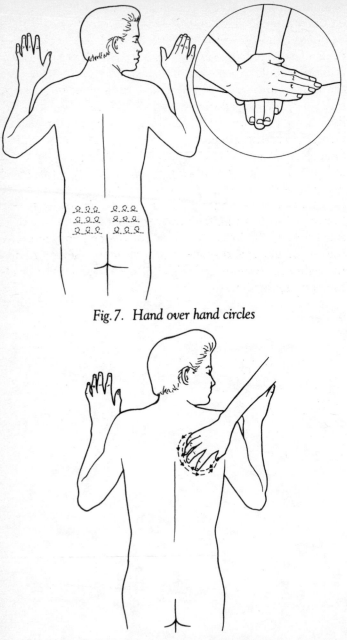

Fig. 7. Hand over hand circles

Fig. 8. Rotating skin on the shoulder blade

your way slowly up to the armpit and back down again. Repeat on the other side (see Fig. 6).

6. Apply some fairly strong pressure to the lower back with the heels of your hands. Put one hand on top of the other and using the whole of your hands work in circles from the base of the spine and over the hips. Then, using your thumbs, work intuitively on any tightness you may find there (see Fig. 7).
7. Repeat the long firm strokes as in Step 1, two or three times.
8. Gently knead the shoulders.
9. Shape your hand as if it were a bird's foot, fingers apart. Place only the fingertips on the shoulder blade. Try to move the skin over the blade in circles. Move several times to the right, then to the left. Repeat on the other shoulder blade (see Fig. 8).
10. Starting from the middle of the back, place your hands side by side horizontally across the spine. Move one hand smoothly to the left shoulder, and at the same time move the other hand to the right hip, stretching the back. Repeat, taking the hands to the opposite hip and shoulder (see Fig. 9).

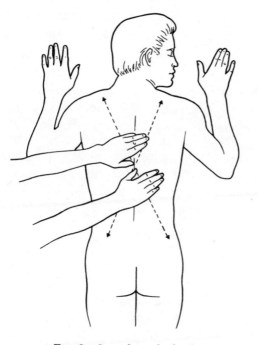

Fig. 9. Stretching the back (1)

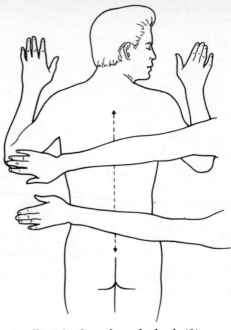

Fig. 10. Stretching the back (2)

11. This time place both your whole forearms horizontally across the back and slide them slowly, yet firmly, apart, one up the back to the top of the shoulders and the other down to the top of the buttocks; use a fair amount of pressure (see Fig. 10).

12. End your massage the same way you began by placing one hand on your partner's head and the other at the base of the spine and then at the feet. When you are ready, move your hands away and cover your partner with a towel. Allow him or her to rest for a while to 'come round' in their own time.

This completes the basic back sequence, but add anything you feel is needed. Work with your whole body, not just your hands and arms. When you are kneading, move gently from side to side in time with your hands. Keep your movements slow and gently flowing. Allow your natural rhythm to come to the fore. Sensitivity at the outset far outweighs a full routine of complicated strokes if they are carried out in a mechanical and impersonal manner. Most of all, develop your own unique style.

The Face and Head

This is an area of the body quite often neglected in remedial massage therapy, yet a good face and scalp massage can be one of the most uplifting experiences of all time. A violent headache can be safely dissolved within minutes without having to resort to aspirin or paracetamol with their accompanying side-effects. Drugs do nothing to remove the cause of a headache which more often than not stems from nervous and muscular tension, something aromatherapy massage will gently soothe away.

If the following sequence is carried out with sensitivity, not only will it relieve tension but it will also effectively stimulate clarity of thought. When there is tension in the neck and spine, particularly where they connect to the brain at the base of the skull, blood flow is impeded. A good flow of blood to the head is vital for optimum brain function.

Mix a facial oil suitable for your partner's skin-type taking into account his or her perfume preference. The skin should be clean and free of make-up. Put two teaspoonfuls of the oil into a saucer; only extremely dry skin will need more than this. Ask your partner to remove spectacles, earrings, necklaces or anything that may impede the massage.

Your partner should be lying down on his or her back *with a cushion or rolled up towel under the knees* to prevent any strain in the lumbar region. The shoulders should be free of clothing. Cover your partner with a thick towel to keep him or her warm. If you are working on the floor, sit cross-legged if possible or kneel on a mat. It is important for you to be comfortable as any tension will be perceived by your partner.

The Face

1. Before you oil your hands, place them on either side of your partner's head. The heels of your hands should cover the forehead, fingers extending downwards anchoring the sides of the head. Hold them there for a few moments (see Fig. 11).
2. Move your hands to the forehead and smoothly stroke the brow, hand-over-hand up and over the hair to the crown of the head. Repeat several times.

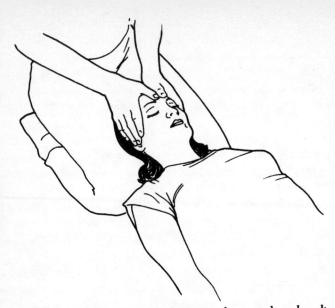

Fig. 11. 'Holding' position for giving face, neck and scalp massage

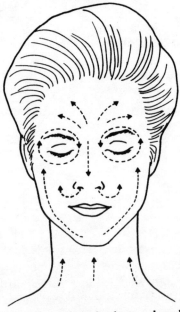

Fig. 12. Oiling the face and neck

3. Move your hands gently away and dip your fingers into the oil. Rub it into your hands. You will need only a smear of oil for the face; if you drench the skin, oil is liable to seep into your partners eyes.

4. Gently slide your hands over your partner's face starting from the chin, circling the eyes and over the forehead. This is simply to oil the skin before you begin the massage (see Fig. 12).

5. Oil your hands a little more generously this time and slide them over the shoulders and up the back of the neck. Go *very* lightly over the throat. Your movements should always be slow and flowing, not brisk and jerky. Use light to medium pressure to avoid dragging the skin, and be particularly careful around the eye area.

6. Place the ball of your thumbs at the centre of the forehead between the eyebrows. Slide both thumbs apart and, when you reach the temples, finish with a little circular flourish before gliding off at the hairline (see Fig. 13).

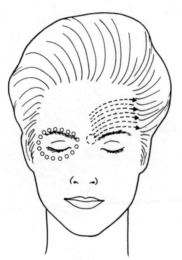

Fig. 13. *Stroking the forehead. Pressure points around the eyes*

7. Return to the starting postion, but this time a little higher up. Repeat Step 6 and continue, a strip at a time, all the way up the forehead until you reach the hairline (see Fig. 13).

8. Place your thumbs at the centre between the eyebrows (the 'third eye') and this time slide your thumbs a little more firmly over the brow bone and off the head. Repeat once or twice.

9. Return to the third eye postion and this time press your thumbs down quite firmly (your partner will soon tell you if it is too hard) and hold for about three seconds. Lift your thumbs and place them a little further out along the brow bone and repeat the pressure. Repeat this at intervals until you reach the outer corners of the eyes (see Fig. 13).

10. Place your forefinger on the body ridge *under* the eyes at the inner corners and repeat the pressing movements, a little more lightly this time, until you reach the outer corner. This is helpful to those who suffer from catarrh or sinus congestion.

Caution: Do not apply pressure if the sinuses are swollen and painful (see Fig. 13).

11. Now allow your partner to bathe in darkness for a few moments. Place your hands gently over the eyes, the heels of your hands creating the darkness, with the fingers extending down over the temples. Keep them there for at least ten seconds (see Fig 14).

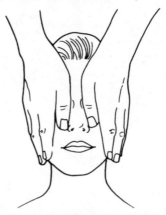

Fig. 14. Bathing in darkness

12. Slide your hands to the sides of your partner's head and apply a little pressure to the temples for about ten seconds.

13. Gently stroke the the entire face with gentle upward movements as in Step 4.

14. Place the ball of your thumbs at the inner corners of the eyes just below the eye-socket. Smooth outwards and upwards towards the temples. Circle the temples as you did in Step 6. Repeat a little lower down, a strip at a time, until you reach the edge of the cheekbone. Repeat the same movement again just below the bone, pressing lightly upwards (see Fig. 15).

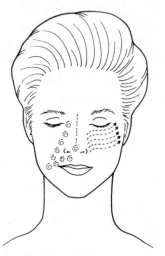

Fig. 15. Stroking and circling the cheeks and nose

15. Place the forefingers on each side of the nose near the bridge. using tiny circles work down the sides of the nose (see Fig. 15).

16. Using your thumbs alternately, stroke down the bridge of the nose from the top to the tip. Circle the tip with the palm of your hand.

17. Using your middle fingers, make tiny circles on the cheeks at either side of the nostrils and over the upper lip (see Fig. 15).

18. Place your thumbs on the chin and pull them slowly and firmly outwards and upwards along the jaw bone to the ear. Repeat a little further inwards until just below the cheek bone (see Fig. 16).

19. Return to the chin and work in tiny circles with your thumbs from the middle of the chin along the jaw bone, finishing behind the ears (see Fig. 16).

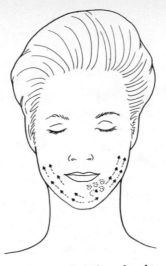

Fig. 16. *Stroking and circling the chin and jaw*

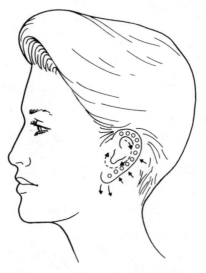

Fig. 17. *Working on the ears*

20. Work in circles behind the ears. Now gently pinch the edges of each ear, working from the top down to the ear lobes. Repeat once or twice, finishing by pulling the ear lobes gently downwards two or three times. Then with the tips of the

forefingers, trace around the spiral of the ears (see Fig. 17).
21. Cup your hands over your partner's eyes as in Step 11.

The Neck

1. Gently turn your partner's head to the left. Place your left hand on his or her forehead or, if you prefer, support the head by letting it rest in your left hand. Place your right hand on your partner's right shoulder and slide your hand firmly all the way up to the neck. When you reach the base of the skull, use all your fingers and gently circle the area several times to release any muscle tension (see Fig. 18).

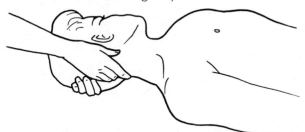

Fig. 18. Stroking and circling the neck

2. Using all your fingers, gently circle the whole right side of the neck. Work from the base of the neck upwards to behind the ears.
3. Repeat the gentle stroking movements, as in Step 2, two or three times.
4. Gently turn your partner's head to the right and repeat Steps 2 to 3 on the left side.
5. Gently move your partner's head to the middle so that he or she is lying straight once more. Place your hands horizontally on the upper chest just under the collar bone, fingers turning inwards towards each other, middle fingertips meeting. Slide your hands away from each other, up and across the shoulders to the back of the neck. Cradle the head in your hands, fingertips meeting.
6. Without stopping, lift your partner's head several centimetres from the floor or table and pull from the base of the skull towards you giving the neck a good stretch. Gently slide your hands up the back of the skull as you allow his or head to come back down gently. Repeat two or three times (see Fig. 19).

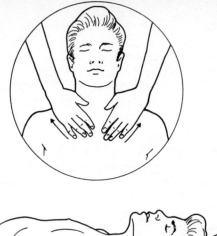

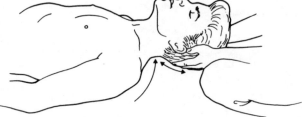

Fig. 19. *Stretching the neck*

The Scalp

Unless your partner is completely bald there is no need to oil the scalp.

1. Lift your partner's head and turn it to the left (see Fig. 20). Using your fingers, press quite firmly and move fingers *and* scalp over the bone. Try not to simply slide your fingers through the hair over the scalp. Work up and down the head covering the entire area. Repeat on the other side and move the head back to the centre.

2. Run your fingers through your partner's hair several times, allowing your fingers to brush the scalp.

3. Finish the entire face, neck and scalp sequence by holding your palms lightly against your partner's forehead with your fingers extending down the temples, as in Fig 11. Hold your hands in this position for a few moments, then gently move them away.

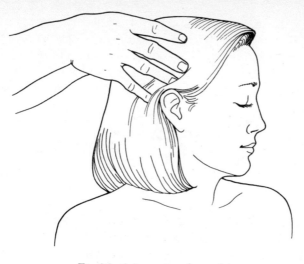

Fig.20. Massaging the scalp

A HEALING TECHNIQUE FOR ALLEVIATING PAIN

If your partner is suffering from aching muscles and joints which the massage may not have completely soothed, try the following technique which can be amazingly pain relieving and balancing to the emotions. Gently 'feather' over the painful spot. That is, with fingers separated, hands very relaxed, *lightly* brush your fingertips downwards over the area several times. Then proceed to sweep over the entire body from head to toes. On reaching the toes, take your hands back to the head and sweep downwards again. Do this about twelve times with rhythmic, flowing movements. Next, lift your hands several centimetres *above* your partner's body and continue with the same sweeping movements, though this time you will be working on the *etheric body*. Finish the sequence by 'holding' – hold the feet for about 30 seconds, then the knees, the hands and finally the head and abdomen: place one hand on your partner's forehead, the other lightly on the abdomen. This will 'ground' your partner, or put him or her back in touch with their physical body. You could use this technique at the start and at the end of *every* massage if you wish and if it feels right for you.

However, if you intend to work at this 'subtle' level all the time, it may be helpful to learn one or two 'psychic protection' techniques (see Chapter 7). It is surprisingly easy to pick up the physical tension and the negative emotions of others if you are at all sensitive. Therefore, you will need to learn how to quickly shake off any uncomfortable feelings, otherwise you will drain your own energy.

SELF-MASSAGE

The ideal situation is to be able to receive a professional aromatherapy massage about once a month, or to have a willing friend with whom to exchange massage. The reality is that few of you will be as fortunate. However, you can still derive much benefit from self-massage with essential oils – though you will, of course, miss out on the deep relaxation engendered by receiving a good massage.

It is best to apply the oils after a warm bath or shower because they will penetrate the skin more readily if it is slightly warm and damp. The direction of your movements should always be towards the heart to encourage a good flow of blood, and therefore nutrients, to the part being treated. Stroke the skin hand-over-hand in an upward direction. Begin with very light strokes and gradually let them become firmer. Once you have improved the circulation, you can begin to knead the fleshy areas of your body such as thighs and calves. When you reach the abdomen, gently circle the area in a clockwise direction to aid peristalsis (waves of muscular contractions which move food through the intestines). This helps to prevent constipation. Finish the massage the way you began with the hand-over-hand stroking.

Self-massage with essential oils, combined with skin-brushing (described at the beginning of this chapter) and aromatic baths will increase your energy levels and bring about a sense of well-being – almost equivalent to a professional aromatherapy massage!

AROMATHERAPY VERSUS CELLULITE

You may be wondering why so much space has been devoted to cellulite in this chapter. Surely, you may be asking, essential oils and tough massage will eventually break it down? Unfortunately, as so may women have discovered, it is not as simple as that. Essential oils, expensive patent 'cures', anti-cellulite creams and tough massage *alone* cannot shift cellulite – especially that which has been in the hips and thighs for many years. As is usual in holistic, or whole person healing, we need to deal with the problem from the *inside* first; this way we may begin to tackle the cause. First, however, let us ask ourselves, what is cellulite and what causes it? Then we can look to the remedy.

If we are to believe the British and American medical establishment, cellulite does not exist; it is simply a fancy French word for fat. Yet in France, doctors take the question of cellulite very seriously indeed. To them, and to all women who suffer from cellulite, it is real enough.

Cellulite is a peculiarly female problem in which the hormone oestrogen plays a part. It is characterised by unsightly lumps and bumps which collect in the thighs, buttocks, hips and upper arms. If the area is pinched the skin puckers and ripples and does not spring immediately back into place. The affected areas look like orange-peel and are cold to the touch. This is because the underlying tissues (unlike ordinary fat) are saturated with water and stagnant wastes.

Cellulite is always more severe in women who lead far from healthy life-styles. That is, if they smoke, get little exercise, overload their digestive systems with junk-food and drink gallons of strong tea or coffee. The contraceptive pill is also a contributing factor. As a result of this onslaught, the lymphatic system fails to cope efficiently with its job of shifting the body wastes to the organs of elimination – the skin, lungs, kidneys and colon. Some of it gets left behind. Then oestrogen comes into play: it acts to protect the vital organs from the rubbish circulating in the blood and lymph by sending the toxins to areas where they will be relatively harmless to a growing baby. In case you are wondering, men too suffer from toxic overload, but instead of getting cellulite, they get furred-up arteries and heart disease. Women, it seems, are protected by biology – that is, until they reach the menopause. After this time, they too are prone to heart attacks because they no longer have the protection of oestrogen in their bodies.

It may be realistic to suggest that a certain amount of cellulite is to be expected in women, but severe cases should be taken seriously.

Indeed, French doctors believe that if left untreated (and they have been treating women with cellulite for forty years) it can lead to serious disorders such as arthritis.

The anti-cellulite programme (as advocated by many aromatherapists and others in the field of natural healing) consists of four main elements: Diet, Dry Skin Brushing, Essential Oils and Lymphatic Drainage Massage. Let us take a look at each one in turn.

Diet

Unfortunately there is not enough space in this book to go into the diet in any detail. However, if you are unable to seek professional help, do read one of the following really excellent books which will tell you everything you will ever need to know about healing through diet: Leslie Kenton's *Biogenic Diet* and Celia Wright's *The Wright Diet*.

Briefly, the diet consists of an initial one or two day fruit 'fast', followed by two weeks on raw fruits and vegetables, nuts, seeds, springwater, juices and herb teas. Thereafter, you adopt a wholefood diet with a little or no dairy products and no more than one cup of coffee or two cups of tea a day. I am afraid it is tough (at least at the beginning), as are all restricted diets, but I promise you, it does work! Incidentally, you will be very pleased to hear that (according to British nutritionist Celia Wright) for *one* day a week you can and *should* feast. Eat anything you like – yes, anything – chocolate, cream, fizzy drinks, coffee. This acts to surprise the liver into activity, for it has very little work to do when you are on a pure diet.

Dry Skin Brushing

Carry out this activity according to the instructions on page 72.

Important: It is best to carry out anti-cellulite treatments either first thing in the morning or, if more convenient, early evening before your evening meal. If you do them last thing at night you might find it difficult to get off to sleep. The combination of skin-brushing, bath and massage is extremely stimulating.

Essential Oils

The oils used for treating cellulite are those which are detoxifying (juniper, lemon) or stimulating for the circulation (cypress, rosemary). They should be used neat in the bath (instructions on page 104) and diluted in vegetable oil for the massage (see recipe page 64). As you lie in the water, knead and pummel the cellulite-laden areas.

Important: Remember not to use the same essence throughout the programme. Like skin-brushing, the body may fail to respond to the same oil if used for longer than three to four weeks continuously.

Example Programme: Weeks 1–3 (juniper), Week 4 (rest), Weeks 5–7 (lemon), Week 8 (rest), Weeks 9–11 (juniper) and so on.

Lymphatic Drainage Massage

It is beyond the scope of this book to describe authentic lymphatic drainage massage as practised by professionals. However, if you are carrying out skin-brushing (which does almost the same job), the following simple self-massage sequence will be extremely beneficial and should be regarded as an important ally in any campaign against cellulite.

Self-Massage for Cellulite

This is best carried out after the skin-brushing and aromatic bath routine. Unlike the gentle technique described earlier, anti-cellulite massage should be vigorous to help drain away toxic wastes from the tissues. You need only a little of your anti-cellulite massage oil – about a teaspoonful for each leg. If you over-oil the skin it will be too slippery to enable you to build up the necessary friction.

1. Using both hands, starting from the ankle, work up to the knee and thigh (front and back) with light stroking, gradually becoming firmer and brisker until you are working quite vigorously (see Fig. 21).

   You can apply the oil to the buttocks if you like, but if you find vigorous massage too awkward to carry out here, there is no need to worry. In most cases, working on the legs and thighs alone shifts cellulite from the surrounding areas because lymphatic drainage is very much increased all-round.

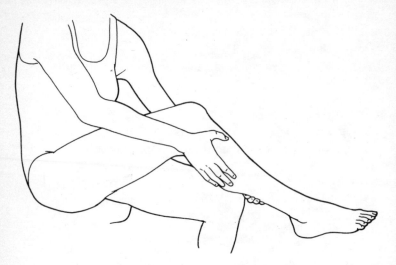

Fig.21. Self-massage for cellulite. Stroking

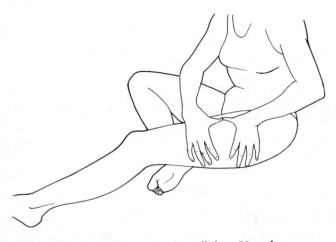

Fig.22. Self-massage for cellulite. Kneading

2. By now you will have stimulated the circulation enough to move on to the next stage, which is kneading. For this you have to pretend you are kneading bread. As you pick up the flesh, squeeze

it and apply as much pressure as you can tolerate, but not so much that you bruise the area. As you continue to knead, using the pads of your thumbs, press firmly into the thighs and hips making small circles all over the area (see Fig 22).

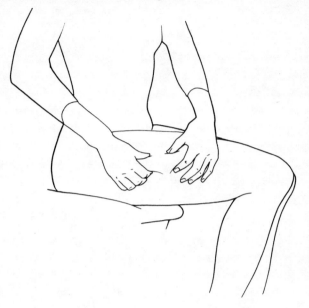

Fig. 23. Self-massage for cellulite. Rolling

3. Next comes rolling. Here you pick up 2 to 3 centimetres of flesh on the thigh and roll it between your fingers and thumb (Fig 23). This helps to break down the pockets of cellulite, thus releasing the toxins into the circulatory systems from which they can be eliminated.
4. Finish off with the long, stroking movements with which you began in Step 1.

After about four or five months on the anti-cellulite programme you will see a dramatic improvement in your figure. You can then reduce the skin-brushing to two or three times a week and the massage to once or twice a week. Continue to use the essential oils in your bath, remembering to alternate between two or three different anti-cellulite essences. However, the healthy eating pattern needs to be a way of life if you are to banish cellulite for good!

OTHER WAYS WITH ESSENTIAL OILS

Let us continue with some more ways of using essential oils for health and pleasure. Remember to refer to the Therapeutic Charts and information on blending as outlined in Chapter 5.

Baths

Essences can be added to your bath simply for pleasure, to aid restful sleep, to help skin disorders, relieve muscular and other pains or to uplift your spirits. They may be used singly or blended with others.

Shake 5 to 10 drops of neat essential oil onto the surface of the water *after* after you have drawn the bath; agitate the water to disperse the oil. If you add essential oils as the water is running, much of the aromatic vapour will have evaporated before you enter the bath. If you have dry skin, you may wish to mix the essences with a few teaspoonfuls of vegetable oil; that is, if you do not mind cleaning a greasy bath afterwards! For a more soluble preparation mix the usual amount of essential oil into a tablespoonful of unperfumed liquid soap.

Foot/Hand Baths

These can be used to ward off chills; for rheumatic or arthritic pain, excessive perspiration, athlete's foot and other skin disorders of the feet or hands such as dermatitis or eczema.

Sprinkle 5 to 6 drops of essential oil (diluted in vegetable oil if desired) to a bowl of hand-hot water and steep feet (or hands) for about 10 minutes. Dry them thoroughly and massage into the skin a a little vegetable oil (or cream) containing a few drops of the same essence(s).

Inhalations

These can be used for colds, 'flu, sinusitis, coughs and as a facial steam treatment (page 76). The simplest method is to add five or six drops of essential oil onto a handkerchief and inhale as required. A few drops of the appropriate oil can be sprinkled onto your pillow to ease nasal congestion and to aid restful sleep.

Steam inhalations should be avoided if you suffer from asthma, as the concentrated steam may trigger an attack, but they can be used to help other respiratory problems such as those mentioned above.

Pour about half a litre of near-boiling water into a bowl and add two to four drops of essential oil. The quantity depends on the strength of the essence. Peppermint, for example, is extremely powerful, whereas sandalwood is very mild. Inhale the vapours for about five minutes, but no longer than ten. To trap the aromatic steam more efficiently, drape a towel over your head and the bowl to make a tent.

Compresses

A compress is a valuable way of treating muscular pain, sprains and bruises as well as reducing pain and congestion in internal organs. The compresses can be used hot or cold according to the condition being treated.

For *recent* injuries such as sprains, bruises, swellings, inflammation and headaches, *cold* compresses are recommended. In the following conditions, *hot* compresses are indicated: old injuries, muscular pain, toothache, menstrual cramp, cystitis, boils, abscesses and so forth.

To make a hot compress, sprinkle about 6 drops of essential oil to about half a litre of water, as hot as you can bear. Place a small towel or a piece of lint or soft fabric on top of the water. Wring out the excess and place the fabric over the area to be treated. Cover this with a piece of 'clingfilm', then lightly bandage in place if necessary; for an ankle or knee for example. Leave the compress in place until it has cooled to body temperature; renew at intervals as required.

For a cold compress, use exactly the same method, but with icy cold water. Leave it in place until it warms to body heat and renew it as required.

Perfuming Rooms

The best way to perfume a room is to use a purpose-designed essential oil burner. These are now widely available from essential oil suppliers (see page 126). However, a drop or two on a pad of *wet* cotton wool or handkerchief will subtly perfume a room if placed on a radiator. An alternative method is to put a drop or two on a light bulb, so that the oil slowly evaporates into the room with the heat of the bulb. Always put the oil onto a *cold* bulb before turning on the light.

A few drops of essential oil can be sprayed around the home using either an atomiser or simple plant spray. Add five drops to 145 ml of water and shake well before use. The effect, however, is short-lived compared to the other methods.

Essential oils can be sprayed around the sick room to prevent the spread of infection during epidemics. The most powerful essences against air-borne bacteria are: pine, thyme, peppermint, lavender, lemon, rosemary, cloves, cinnamon, eucalyptus and tea tree. Eucalyptus and tea tree oils are credited with anti-viral properties as well and are useful as a room fumigant should a member of the family be stricken with 'flu.

Skin Perfumes

Essential oils can be used alone or blended with other essences to make delightful perfumes. They may be used purely for pleasure or to back-up the healing potential of other aromatherapy treatments – particularly helpful for stress-related problems. For the occasional attack of anxiety or depression, as is most common, essential oils will certainly lift your spirits. When anxiety or depression becomes a way of life, however, it would be advisable to seek the help of a professional aromatherapist or other holistic therapist.

7

On Becoming Whole

PLATO'S WORDS of wisdom echo down the centuries:

The cure of the part should not be attempted without treatment of the whole, and also no attempt should be made to cure the body without the soul, and therefore if the head and body are to be well you must begin by curing the mind: that is the first thing. . . . For this is the error of our day in the treatment of the human body, that physicians separate the soul from the body.

Plato, *Chronicles*

Even though Plato wrote these words over two thousand years ago, we in the modern western world are only just beginning to resonate in harmony with his tune of truth. Our eyes have been closed for many centuries, yet the sages and physicians of the East have never lost sight of the reality of the WHOLE. In our newfound realisation, we have coined the word *holistic* to summarise this concept.

The word *holistic* has its roots in the Greek *holos* which means 'whole'. In holistic healing, the whole person – mind-body-spirit – is taken into account. In all schools of natural healing, which includes aromatherapy, the most important underlying principle is that the body will heal itself if given the chance. This is achieved by sound nutrition, adequate exercise, fresh air and sunshine, and above all, by seeking the ways in which we may find inner contentment. Body, mind and spirit are interrelated; whatever affects one aspect will affect the whole.

In this chapter, I shall attempt to separate the parts that make up the whole, then to explore some of the ways in which we may bring about harmony to mind-body-spirit.

MIND

Even in orthodox circles, the idea that our state of mind and personality has an influence over our physical health is beginning to gain credence once again. For instance, there is a so-called 'cancer personality'. Such people give more than they take; they tend to hide their emotions and repress their desires just to please others. The 'migraine personality' is driven by guilt. These people are perfectionists, ambitious, hard-working and extremely neat and tidy. The 'eczema personality' is hypersensitive and, like the cancer type, tends to repress his or her emotions. The 'heart-attack personality', on the other hand, is aggressive, impatient, competitive and ambitious.

The great psychologist Carl Jung has written about the 'symbolism of illness'. He says that the *form* which an illness takes can be a reflection of the mental state. He cites examples of nausea with no apparent cause, where the patient is unconsciously saying 'I'm sick of this situation'. Another patient with inexplicable leg pains is saying 'I can't stand any more'.

In a wider sense, we need to consider the effects of world issues such as damage to the environment by pollution of air, soil and water; the rapidly diminishing rain forests; wars, faminine, and the nuclear threat. All of these issues can be a source of great emotional turmoil to many people.

The pressures of being poor, disabled, black, unemployed, or whatever, can lead to feelings of frustration, anger, resentment and depression. Such feelings almost inevitably lead to physical illness.

Almost all of us can recall a time in our lives when we have been under emotional stress and have become ill as a result. Perhaps it was just a cold, or possibly something more serious. Many people also become more accident-prone at such times.

Before we go any further we need to define what we mean by stress. Most people think of stress as the outside pressures and problems that impinge upon them. Problems such as deadlines, noise, marital strife, excessive demands made on our time by others, and so forth. In actual fact, stress is our own personal reaction to those things (or people) 'out there'. Some people, for instance, cannot sleep if there is traffic noise at night; others hardly notice it and may even welcome it as a 'sign of life' (I have heard this said more than once!) While one person may have a nervous breakdown as a result of financial pressures or divorce, another may react quite differently. They may grieve or worry for a while, but will work towards improving their situation, first by acceptance, and eventually coming to view the set-back as an impetus for change and growth.

While a certain amount of stress can be positive – it provides energy which enables us to do the things we want to do – it only becomes a problem if it develops into *distress*. This means we begin to develop symptoms which can lead to illness.

Conversely, it is possible for our *physical* state to influence our moods, behaviour patterns and, in extreme cases, our sanity. Certain forms of schizophrenia, for instance, can be triggered by food allergies to substances such as wheat gluten, caffeine, alcohol and chemical food additives. This leads us into the next stage of whole-healing, namely diet.

BODY

Let food be your medicine, and medicine your food.

Hippocrates

Food is an emotive subject; so many arguments rage as to what constitutes the 'ideal diet'. Is meat good for us? Should we be vegetarian or even vegan? Or is the macrobiotic principle the ideal? My response to such questions is to suggest that there is no one ideal diet suitable for everyone. We are each very different with varying needs. Whatever we may believe about diet, the only clear-cut 'rule', as far as I see it, is that our food should be as free as possible from harmful additives and the toxic residues of modern farming methods – no easy task nowadays.

It may be relatively easy to buy organically grown flour, but unsprayed organically grown fruit and vegetables are a rarity – unless you are able to grow them yourself. Even when they are available they can be expensive, prohibitively so for some people. The best we can do at the moment, until the 'organic revolution' hits the high street, is to eat foods as near as possible to their natural state – not out of tins and packets.

It is beyond the scope of this book to go into dietary reform in any detail, but the following steps outline a wholefood diet as recommended by many aware nutritionists. It does not take into account food allergies – some people are allergic to wheat for example – or if you wish to avoid animal foods altogether (veganism) or whether, like myself, you prefer not to eat meat or fish. It should, however, serve as a useful guide that can be adapted to suit individual needs. Aim to alter your diet *gradually* over a period of six months. Drastic overnight changes will certainly lead to digestive upsets. For those wishing to go deeper, I have suggested two excellent books on healing through diet (page 129).

1. Buy organically grown food if you can, but do not fret if you cannot (which will only cause stress).
2. Eat more wholemeal bread and other high-fibre foods such as dried beans, lentils, nuts, oats, brown rice and other wholegrain cereals.
3. Eat plenty of fresh fruit and vegetables – preferably unskinned, well scrubbed and raw in salads or lightly cooked.
4. Cut down on all fats, particularly those from animal sources especially lard, suet, double cream and full-fat cheeses. Use moderate amounts of cold-pressed vegetable oils such as virgin olive, sesame and sunflowerseed.
5. Sweeten your food sparingly with honey, or more lavishly with dried fruits such as dates, figs, sultanas and raisins.
6. Cut down on salt and use more herbs to flavour your food.
7. Buy free-range eggs if possible.
8. Eat red meat only once a week (if at all). Instead, eat more fish, particularly oily fish such as mackerel.
9. Cut down on milk. Try using skimmed or semi-skimmed milk, or substitute dairy milk with soya milk.
10. Try to avoid processed foods in cans and packets – especially those laden with chemical additives. These foods should only be eaten occasionally; they should not form the basis of your diet.
11. Drink plenty of water (bottled or filtered), herb teas, diluted fruit juices, and only one or two cups of ordinary tea or coffee a day if you cannot give it up altogether.

12. Eat slowly in convivial surroundings and, above all, enjoy your food.

MOVEMENT

The human body was designed to move. Unlike a machine that breaks down with use, we become stronger, more flexible and age more slowly if every muscle and joint is used frequently.

When we lived a simpler life we walked, swam, stretched and climbed as a matter of course almost every day of our lives. We did not consciously 'exercise', nor did we require supplementary exercise to keep our bodies finely tuned.

In relation to stress, regular exercise increases the circulation which in turn increases oxygen levels in the blood and activates the hormonal system (the endocrine glands). This has a definite positive effect on our state of mind. Anyone who has recently taken up some form of exercise will tell that it has brought them enhanced mental energy and concentration, the ability to sleep more deeply and a feeling of well-being.

Natural movement which is also a pleasure rather than a chore is infinitely superior to indoor exercises with weights, or exercise that is so taxing that one aches from head to toe afterwards. Jogging is not a particularly good form of exercise (especially on city pavements); all that pounding can put a great deal of strain on the lower back and can damage the knees. Why not swim, dance, walk in the country or go rowing, canoeing or hill climbing, or anything else that you *enjoy* doing, as long as you use your body efficiently.

If you are elderly, physically disabled or too ill to take vigorous exercise, do not despair: regular aromatherapy massage and/or dry skin brushing (see Chapter 6) can be almost as beneficial.

LIGHT

Natural light is as much a nutrient as food and water. It is absorbed by our bodies and used in a wide range of metabolic processes. Light affects the body in two ways: directly (tanning and the formation of vitamin D from ergosterol) and indirectly through the photoreceptors in our eyes. The photoreceptors are part of a nerve network which lead directly to the brain. The type and quality of light can affect our hormonal balance and body chemistry as a whole, influencing our energy levels and the way we feel. The most common problems associated with light deprivation (experienced by indoor workers) are lethargy, headaches, irritability, lack of concentration and a seasonal mental state known as 'winter depression'.

The morning rays are said by yogis to be highly charged with *prana* (life-force) and are the most beneficial to health. In any case, the longer waves of ultra-violet light before noon (and also after four in the afternoon) are less likely to burn. So, if you enjoy sunbathing, a couple of hours first thing, or very late in the day will be better for your skin. Bear in mind however, that a little of the sun's powerful energy is good, but too much can result in premature ageing – or even skin cancer.

FRESH AIR

Air is so vital that it is only possible to live for a few minutes without it. We all know how essential oxygen is for the lungs and the whole organism, but few of us remember that the skin also needs air as a stimulus for its normal functioning. For this reason, it has been referred to a 'the third lung'. You may have heard the horrific tale of the small boy who was painted from head to toe with a metallic-based substance for a carnival and who consequently died of respiratory failure.

Most people cover their bodies with layers of synthetic fibres that trap air and hinder the skin's natural metabolism. Clothes should ideally be of cotton and other natural fibres such as linen and wool, as they allow perspiration to evaporate by the free-flow of air they afford.

Whenever possible (especially if you live in a large town or city), visit the seaside and breathe in the bracing sea air. It is charged with negative ions which generate a feeling of well-being. The clean, crisp air of mountainous regions is perhaps the most beneficial of all. If you live far from the sea and mountains, do not underestimate the value of your local park. Take a daily walk in the park and breathe deeply. These precious moments of breathing in the scents of grass, trees and flowers will help to bring about a state of harmony to a bustling mind and jangled nervous system.

SPIRIT

One way of defining the spiritual aspect of 'self' is to say it is our purpose for living. Without purpose, we become depressed or apathetic; life then appears bleak and meaningless. Even when we do not follow a conscious spiritual path in terms of a religious faith, we may in fact be realising our purpose in some other way. It could be through an art-form or simply by a love of nature. Or more actively perhaps, by working towards the realisation of a humanitarian ideal.

MIND-BODY-SPIRIT

If you are experiencing difficulty in any of the key areas of life listed below, the chances are that you are not experiencing whole health. All of these aspects are interrelated and, as such, are not listed in any order of importance, nor is this list in any way comprehensive.

1. Eating and drinking: under-eating, over-eating, poor diet in general for whatever reason – choice, ignorance, poverty.
2. Breathing: polluted air, poor posture, smoking.
3. Elimination: problems may manifest as constipation, fluid retention, congested skin, catarrh.
4. Personal hygiene.
5. Ecological and political: frustration, anger, despair.
6. Mobility: problems experienced by elderly or disabled people.
7. Controlling body temperature: problems of the elderly and the very young.
8. Communicating: problems experienced by handicapped people or those suffering from lack of confidence or a speech impediment.
9. Work: unemployment, stressful work, boredom.
10. Relationships: marriage, family, friends, workmates, loneliness.
11. Sexuality: problems of acceptance experienced by gays and lesbians: psychological problems as a result of incest or rape.
12. Money: poverty, debt, greed.
13. Feelings of inequality: being female, black, divorced, a single

parent, dissatisfied with appearance, physical/ mental handicap, etc.

14. Play: no recreation/fun in life.
15. Freedom: imprisonment (jail), living under an oppressive regime.
16. Creativity/spirituality: no outlet for artistic expression, religious beliefs, humanitarian ideals.
17. Being divorced from nature: inability or unwillingness to see/touch/smell/experience the elements, flowers, trees, or to walk on earth, rock, grass, sand.
18. Sleeping: broken sleep, insomnia, needing to sleep more than 10 hours *every* night, problems associated with shift work.
19. Environment: not only pollution, but dislike of one's surroundings at home or at work etc.
20. Death: fear of dying, inability to face up to the idea of death or bereavement.

TOWARDS INTEGRATION

The following mind-body exercises will help you to get in touch with your inner powers. By creating a peaceful space within your life, you will begin to tap a source of self-healing, an energy that will enable you to become much more in control of life. You will begin to react less self-destructively to 'outside' pressures, becoming stronger and more resourceful in the face of adversity. Never under-estimate the power of the mind-body, which can either trap or liberate the spiritual aspect of self. The condition of spiritual imprisonment or freedom depends on many things, but especially on how we breathe and think. We cannot change our outer situation, but we can change our attitude to it, which makes all the difference in the world.

Breath of Life

Hold your breath for a few moments. Let the breath flow in again and ask yourself 'What is life?'. Could it be breath?

The air we breathe is shared by all life on our planet. By *consciously* breathing, that is, by becoming aware of the breath as it flows in and out, we begin to recognise the pattern of life itself: the ebb and flow of the tides; the waxing and waning of the Moon. Our oneness with the trees (often referred to as the planet's lungs) becomes manifest fact. Even the shape of a tree – with its numerous branches and twigs – resembles the general outline of our own lungs.

As breathing is the only one of the body's functions that can be either voluntary or involuntary, it can form a bridge between the conscious and the unconscious. In other words, by influencing our breathing, we can change our energy levels and our mood.

Many of us are shallow breathers; we use only the upper part of our lungs, which means that toxic residues are not completely removed. As a result, the blood is deprived of much of the oxygen it needs to feed the body tissues, so we may end up feeling listless or suffer vagueness of thought. At the same time, the oxygen deficit hinders the assimilation of nutrients from the food we eat.

The Complete Breath

The yoga 'complete breath' is one of the easiest ways to begin learning to use your lungs efficiently and is very helpful to those suffering from respiratory ailments such as asthma, bronchitis and so forth. Furthermore, by learning to breathe properly, we begin to strengthen the aura (see page 119), or the body's immune system if you prefer to think of it in more material terms. The 'Complete Breath' exercise (and the one which follows after) is best performed outside in the fresh air if possible, at least three times a week. The next best place is a well-ventilated room. You could enhance the experience (and deepen your breathing) by vaporising any of the following 'respiratory' essences into the room: myrrh, frankincense, pine-needle, cedarwood, juniper, cypress. You may have noticed they are all tree oils! Use a purpose designed essential oil burner/vaporiser or try one of the other methods as suggested in Chapter 6.

1. Lie on a rug on the floor or ground if outside (in a garden perhaps), or on a firm bed with your arms at your sides, several centimetres away from your body, palms face down.
2. Close your eyes and begin to inhale through your nose very slowly. Expand your abdomen slightly, then pull the air up into the rib-cage, and then your chest. Your abdomen will be automatically drawn in as the ribs move out and the chest expands. Hold for a few seconds.

3. Now begin to breathe out slowly through your nose in a smooth continuous flow until the abdomen is drawn in and the rib-cage and chest are relaxed. Hold for a few seconds before repeating two or three times.
4. Now breathe in slowly as you did in Step 1 but gradually raise your arms overhead in time with the inhalation until the backs of your hands touch the floor.
5. Hold your breath for ten seconds while you have a good stretch.
6. Slowly breathe out as you bring your arms back down to your sides. Repeat two or three times (see Fig. 24).

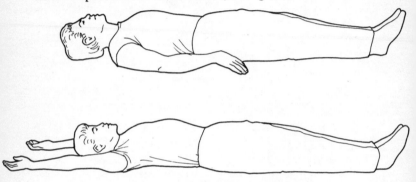

Fig. 24. *The Complete Breath.*
Breathe deeply without strain (steps 1–3).
Breathe in and raise arms overhead. Bring arms back down
to side on the out-breath (steps 4–6).

Flight

To experience an exhilarating feeling of flight, imagine you are about to soar up into the clouds as your arms are thrust forward and backward in rhythmic motion. If performed correctly (see Fig. 25) with synchronised breathing, this movement will loosen a stiff back and shoulders, and at the same time, encourage you to breathe more fully.

1. Stand with feet apart, arms outstretched at sides. Close your eyes, inhale and bend back as far as you can (without any discomfort) thrusting your arms back. Hold for five seconds.
2. Exhale, bend forward and down, keeping arms back and up, but keep your neck limp. Hold for five seconds. Inhale and bend back again. Repeat the same movements three times, increasing

the backward and forward stretches as you become warmer and therefore more flexible.

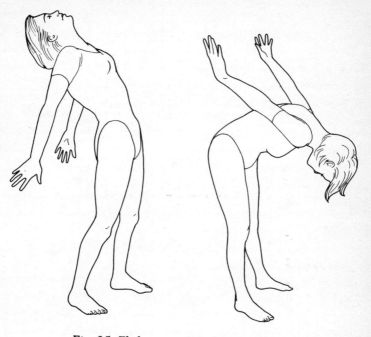

Fig. 25 Flight   Step 1   Step 2

Deep Relaxation

Regular relaxation and meditation should become part of our lives, especially if we live far from nature in a fuzz of constant activity, forever striving to meet deadlines.

Before attempting the meditation and visualisation exercises suggested later in this chapter, it is important to master the art of letting go. This will greatly enhance your ability to concentrate, to meditate and to visualise – an important adjunct in self-healing and when giving healing massage.

There are numerous relaxation techniques taught by experts in the field of 'stress management'. The technique outlined below is known as *progressive muscular relaxation* and is one of the easiest to master. The idea is to become aware of the two extremes of tension and release, for until we do a thing consciously, we are not fully

117

aware of it. Awareness is the key to letting go. The act of tensing, stretching and releasing is also extremely satisfying to practise.

Find a quiet, well-ventilated room with pleasant surroundings if possible, where you will not be disturbed for at least fifteen minutes. Clothing should be loose and comfortable; take off your shoes. To enhance the atmosphere, vaporise your favourite relaxing essential oil(s). If you live in a noisy area, it may also be helpful to play a tape of gentle music.

1. Lie down on the floor or on a firm bed supported by pillows if desired – one under your head and another under your knees which will support your lower back.
2. Close your eyes, take one or two deep breaths and let out the air with a deep sigh.
3. Now become aware of your feet. As you inhale, tighten them, curling your toes under then flexing them towards your body. Hold on to this tension for a slow count to five, then let your feet relax and become limp as you breathe out with a sigh.
4. As you inhale, think of your calves and tense them as you count slowly to five, holding onto the tension. Now let go of the tension as you breathe out with a sigh of relief.
5. Progress to your knees, then your thighs, buttocks, abdomen, chest, shoulders, hands, arms, neck, head and face. Tense each part then let it go, experiencing a wonderful sensation of release.
6. Take three deep breaths, breathing in as far as you can but without straining. Hold the breath for a moment then slowly exhale.
7. Now become aware of your body and 'feel' around for any areas that still feel tense and repeat the tightening and releasing of the muscles until you feel deeply relaxed and at peace.
8. When you feel ready (after at least five minutes of lying quietly and breathing normally) have a good stretch from fingertips to toes before slowly getting up.

Important: This relaxation exercise is most beneficial if practised once or twice a day on an empty stomach, or at least an hour after eating.

Once you have become accustomed to the idea of conscious relaxation (as in the previous exercise), you will eventually progress to the stage whereby the relaxation response is triggered by a simple action and/or silent prompt. If you feel yourself tensing up, then spare a few moments to release that tension and see the difference it can make. All you have to do while sitting at home or at work, or on a train or bus, is to tense up the arm and leg muscles, then let them go, saying to yourself 'I am relaxed'. Do this if you are nervous before an interview for example, or before facing any difficult situation at work or in your private life. By lessening your own tension you help to relax others in your sphere; relaxation and tension are infectious.

AURIC CONTROL OR 'PSYCHIC PROTECTION'

Before embarking on any form of mental/spiritual development, which includes meditation, it is essential that you are able to understand the function of the aura (see also page 39) and are able to control and strengthen your own aura. This is an excellent discipline because a strong aura will protect you from 'influences' of all kinds – anything from germs to stress.

A healthy aura is rather like a filter, allowing only that which is beneficial to affect us; this is what it *should* achieve in a well-balanced person. However, in a world of much stress and strain, the aura can become weakened, allowing inharmonious influences to enter. This gives rise to mental and physical tensions which can result in illness.

To understand how to control your aura you must first realise that it is largely a thought emanation and as such, can easily be controlled by thought. Close your eyes and imagine that you are centred within a sphere of white light which also permeates your body. Feel that you are protected within this sphere of light (like the yolk within an egg) and that the energy around you is unbroken, especially over your head. Some people prefer to think of blue or golden light; others may not think of a colour at all but just *feel* they are centred within a sphere.

With practice, this visualisation (or feeling) of your auric space will become an automatic process. It can be carried out at any time when you feel the need, for example, when you are near anybody with a cold or 'flu; when you are experiencing any form of fear; when others are indulging in negative emotions; in noisy surroundings; first thing in the morning and last thing at night; after meditating or giving intuitive aromatherapy massage.

While, of course, it is necessary to become sensitive to the needs of others, even if this means taking on a little of their pain *at the time*, it is not good to allow this negativity to linger (remember my experience with Charlotte? – Chapter 3). If we hold on to the suffering of those nearest to us, we may not be strong enough to offer any real help by lifting them from whatever is affecting them. The ability to empathise, to connect with our own and each other's inner strength, is a necessary part of giving healing massage or even when offering a shoulder to cry on. The feeling of empathy is closely linked with our intuitive and higher feelings, whereas sympathy hooks into our personal distress.

As well as thinking of your aura, another way of protecting yourself while giving massage, and without blocking that all-important sensitivity, is to become a *channel* rather than the *source* of healing energies. At the start of the massage close your eyes and visualise (or feel) a source of energy above your head: a ball of white light, or maybe the Sun. As you inhale, imagine you are drawing energy from this source of light, in through the top of your head and out through your hands and feet as you exhale. By seeing yourself open as a chalice, a channel of cosmic energies, you reduce the risk of becoming drained as a result of drawing on your own energy reserves.

The power of thought is everything. In fact, if you are able to do this successfully, and if there is an empathy between yourself and your partner, the experience will be enlivening for both parties.

At the end of the massage 'ground' yourself. That is, become aware of your feet in contact with the ground (best if you are barefoot). Stamp your feet if necessary. It is common to feel light-headed or 'distant' after working intuitively, unless you consciously return to terra-firma. Once you feel grounded, enclose yourself safely within your aura.

Ideally, your partner should be able to 'close down' by thinking of his or her own aura. However, you could send a 'closing thought' to your partner *before* you ground and enclose yourself. Simply visualise or think the person safely enclosed within their own spiritual space.

Water can be used as a protective element. After giving massage, hold your hands under a running tap. If you feel drained (despite having carried out the previous visualisations), take a shower, if possible, or a bath containing essence of juniper. A drop of juniper can also be rubbed into your forearms and solar plexus. Juniper is regarded by many intuitive aromatherapists as having the power to cleanse on a psychic as well as a physical level.

THE BACH FLOWER REMEDIES

The Bach Flower Remedies are prepared from non-poisonous wild flowers – they are benign in their action, non-addictive and can be taken by people of all ages. As well as helping us transmute negative emotions such as anger, fear and hate into optimism and joy, they can be used for psychic protection – and the effect can be immediate. Rescue Remedy (a composite remedy of five different flowers) is indespensable in this respect.

This system of healing was discovered by Edward Bach, a doctor who had practised for over 20 years in London as a consultant, bacteriologist and homoeopath. The late Dr Bach gave up his lucrative pratice in 1930 to seek energies in the plant world which would restore vitality to the sick or distressed.

Dr Bach developed great sensitivity. If he held his hand over a flowering plant, he could sense in himself the healing properties of that flower. In this way he found 38 flowers to cover all known negative states of mind.

The usual method of taking the Bach Remedies is to put a few drops in a cup of springwater which is then sipped at intervals. Bach Flower Remedies are available from many health food shops or they may be obtained by mail order from the Bach Centre in Oxfordshire, England (see page 133).

NATURE ATTUNEMENT

Nature is the most potent source of healing for the mind-body-spirit. An hour's walk in the countryside will dissipate any uncomfortable feelings absorbed from others. Silent contemplation of the sounds of moving water works well for many people. Close your eyes and listen to the music of a running stream, flowing river, waterfall or the waves of the sea. If you live far from any natural source of running water, an ornamental fountain in a park or garden can be of equal value. Or sit for a while with your back against the trunk of a mature tree (preferably an oak); breathe deeply and allow yourself to merge, as it were, with the energies of the tree. Never underestimate the simplicity of this approach. Many of us are cut off from the natural Earth currents, especially when we live in cities. Unknowingly, we become dreadfully out of balance when divorced from the nurture of the living Earth.

FIRST STEPS IN MEDITATION

The type of meditation outlined here is known as REFLECTIVE MEDITATION. Many experts in the field, including the Pegasus Foundation (my own teachers) based in Malvern, England, believe this *active* form of meditation is more suited to the western mind. Many eastern approaches are *passive* in that they aim to empty the mind, or help us to reach the stage whereby we become observers of our own thoughts as if we were somehow separate from them. Reflective meditation, on the other hand, involves thinking about a definite subject, theme, thought or word. This is actually the simplest form of meditation and is best suited to the beginner. Meditation should ideally be practised for fifteen to twenty minutes daily, preferably first thing in the morning. However, even as little as two or three sessions a week can help to reduce stress, improve concentration and encourage creativity and inspiration.

The Dove

1. Sit comfortably in a quiet room or in a garden if you prefer. A crossed legged position may be adopted if you are accustomed to this position, otherwise sit in a straight-backed chair with your feet firmly on the ground and your hands resting loosely in your lap.
2. Close your eyes. Empty your lungs and breathe deeply in through your nose. Do not strain, simply become aware of your breath as it flows in and out.
3. Concentrate on your feet; let them go, thinking relaxation into them. Then go over each part of your body in turn, letting go and relaxing – your calves, knees, thighs, hips, abdomen and chest; your hands, arms, shoulders, neck, face, eyes, brow – even your tongue and scalp.
4. Imagine you are centred within a sphere of light – your aura.

5. Now direct your thoughts to a beautiful white dove. Consider that the bird is of the element air. It possesses the ability to fly whereas you cannot.

6. Hear the coo of the dove, the flap of its wings. Reach out and touch the firm silky feathers of its back, the downy feathers of its breast. Does the presence of the bird instil in you an awareness of its form and beauty?

7. Become as one with the dove . . . you *are* the dove. Open your wings and take flight; rise above your abode – feel the exhilaration of movement through the air . . . the wings of the bird symbolise the ability of the spirit to soar above the mundane. Dive and glide in the blue sky then let the air currents carry you along. Experience the peace, the freedom of flight . . .

8. When you are ready, fly down to Earth; settle on the moist green banks of a running stream. Drink from the crystal waters.

9. Now it is time to shake yourself free from the gentle form of the dove. Separate your consciousness from it . . . watch as it ascends once more – alone. You are yourself again.

10. Direct your consciousness back into your body. Imagine yourself centred along a straight line running from the top of your head to your feet. Feel safely enclosed within your sphere of light.

11. Open your eyes. Shake out your limbs, stamp your feet (to bring you back to terra-firma), have a good stretch. You will feel calm and at peace with the world.

You might like to meditate on any of the following subjects: a lion, a rainbow, the Sun, the Moon, the Earth, a tree, a fish, a flower (of your choice). Follow the same format as with the dove meditation. Carry out the breathing and body consciousness/relaxation (Steps 1 to 4) then direct your attention to the subject. First the intellectual consideration: see the subject clearly in your mind. Note the differences between yourself and the subject. Then the emotional consideration: hear the coo of the dove for example, or smell the perfume of a rose, bask in the warmth of the Sun. The spiritual consideration: in this phase you become identified with the subject of concentration. You are no longer thinking about it because you are it. Finally, disengagement and relaxation: shake yourself free from the form of your subject. See it once more as separate from yourself, then direct your consciousness back into your body as in Steps 9–11.

IN CONCLUSION

It would be unrealistic to suggest that a good organic diet, daily meditation and aromatherapy massage is the answer to life's problems, and that it will somehow cocoon us in an etheric pink haze for the rest of our days! Aromatherapy and the rest cannot solve the problem of congenital disorders such as a leaking heart valve, liver or kidney dysfunction or mental handicap, nor alter the fact that some people are born healthier than others. What these things *can* do is to enhance the quality of life by helping us to transmute 'stress' into positive challenges, thus preventing the onset of apathy or even depression. This will enable us to shake off minor ills and possibly prevent the onset of chronic illness such as heart disease, high blood pressure, diabetes and the many other diseases of civilization.

In a broader sense, people with a calm, positive and compassionate attitude to life are perhaps better equipped to help solve the many ecological, social and political problems facing the world today.

May the art of aromatherapy thrive and bloom and restore our faith in the healing power of aromatic plants – a gift from Gaia, Goddess of the living Earth.

Notes

1. Coleman, Dr V. *A Guide to Alternative Medicine*.
2. Schnaubelt, Dr K. *Oils for Viral Diseases*. International Journal of Aromatherapy.
3. Valnet, Dr J. *The Practice of Aromatherapy*.
4. The Story of John is an abridged version of the account which appeared in The International Journal of Aromatherapy.
5. Dodd, G. and Van Toller, S. *Perfumery*.
6. Maury, M. *The Secret of Life and Youth*.

Toxicity of Essential Oils

Essential oils are safe and extremely beneficial if used sensibly as outlined in this book. Toxicity can occur, however, if large quantities are taken by mouth. Although a few older books on aromatherapy recommend oral doses, most aromatherapists now advise against this practice. Oral doses should only be taken under the guidance of a medical herbalist or clinical aromatherapist.

One or two essences should never be used in therapy. Sasafrass, for example (if you can find it) can cause cancer. Before using any essential oil, please refer to the following check-list.

To be avoided by the layperson: Pennyroyal, thuja, sage (not to be confused with clary-sage which is safe to use), wintergreen, thyme.

Not to be applied to the skin: (these oils are best used as room perfumes): cinnamon bark, cinnamon leaf, cloves.

Not to be applied before sunbathing   (these oils, especially bergamot, may cause temporary pigmentation): bergamot, lemon, orange, mandarin, grapefruit, lime, verbena.

Not to be used in Pregnancy: Basil, myrrh, thyme, marjoram (sweet).

A WORD ABOUT ALLERGIES

It is possible to be allergic to almost anything – even to the seemingly innocuous sweet almond oil. A few people may be skin-sensitive to peppermint, basil, bergamot, ylang-ylang, lemongrass, verbena, ginger or geranium if used in dilutions above 1½ to 2 per cent, more especially if applied to the sensitive skin of the face.

If you are one of the rare people allergic to all essences, unfortunately, you will have to try another therapy such as herbalism or homoeopathy.

Glossary

A guide to explain some of the jargon you may come across in aromatherapy literature and essential oil suppliers' lists.

Absolute: Extracted from plant material, usually flowers, by solvents such as benzene, hexane and petroleum ether.

Aromark Grade Oil: Tested for purity and authenticated by the Essential Oil Trade Association (EOTA). A pure essential oil from a named botanical species from a given country of origin. Usually organically produced from plants grown without the use of poisonous sprays and chemical fertilizers. The label should state whether the oil is organic.

Aromatic Oil: Although I have used the term to describe the nature of essential oils, be wary of a bottle of oil labelled as such: it may be synthetic or a blend of essential oils diluted in vegetable oil, or it may be an infused oil (see below).

Bergamot F.C.F.:   Bergaptene free. Bergaptene can cause skin pigmentation changes when exposed to sunlight.

Carrier/Base Oil: A vegetable oil such as soya, corn or sunflowerseed in which essential oils are diluted for massage.

Essential Oil/Essence/Etheric Oil/Volatile Oil: The odoriferous, volatile (evaporates in the open air) component of an aromatic plant, usually captured by distillation.

Fixed Oil: Ordinary vegetable oil such as soya or corn which does not evaporate in the open air.

Infused Oil: Usually a herbal oil such as comfrey, St John's wort or marigold. Plant material is placed in vegetable oil and heated until the aroma has permeated the oil. It is then strained and used as a massage oil.

Perfume: Usually a blend of synthetic chemicals; it may contain a small amount of essential oil. If labelled 'Natural Perfume' it should contain 100 per cent essential oil and is usually diluted in ethyl alcohol, vegetable oil or wax such as jojoba.

Perfume   Compound/Perfume   Oil/Pot   Pourri   Reviver   Oil: Synthetic.

Resinoid: Extracted from gums and resins by solvents in the same way as an absolute.

Rose Otto: Captured by distillation. Other rose oils such as Rose Maroc Absolute are extracted by solvents.

Ylang-Ylang Extra: This refers to the quality of the oil. Ylang-ylang 1,2,3 and cananga oil is also available. Extra is best (it has a superior aroma) then in diminishing quality: 1,2,3, Cananga. Ylang-ylang Extra is obtained from the 'first running' of the distillation process which continues for the subsequent grades.

Further Reading

Bek, L. and Pullar, P. *The Seven Levels of Healing*, Rider, 1986.

Capra, F. *The Tao of Physics*, Flamingo, 1985.

Chancellor, P.M. *Handbook of the Bach Flower Remedies*, C.W. Daniel, 1971.

Coleman, Dr. V. *Body Power*, Thames and Hudson, 1983.

Coleman, Dr. V. *A Guide to Alternative Medicine*, Corgi, 1988.

Davis, P. *Aromatherapy, an A-Z*, C.W. Daniel, 1989.

Dodd, G and Van Toller, S. *Perfumery*, Chapman and Hall, 1988.

Downing, G. *The Massage Book*, Penguin Books, 1972.

Griggs, B. *Green Pharmacy*, Jill Norman and Hobhouse, 1982.

Hodgkinson, L. *How to Banish Cellulite Forever*, Grafton, 1989.

Hoffmann, D. *The New Holistic Herbal*, Element Books, 1989.

Kenton, L. *The Biogenic Diet*, Century Arrow, 1986.

Maury, M. *The Secret of Life and Youth*, C.W. Daniel, 1989.

Maxwell-Hudson, C., foreword by. *The Book of Massage*, Ebury, 1984.

Ryman, D. *The Aromatherapy Handbook*, Century, 1984.

Schnaubelt, Dr K. *Oils for Viral Diseases*, International Journal of Aromatherapy, Winter 1988/Spring 1989.

Tansley, D. *The Rainment of Light*, Routledge and Keegan Paul, 1985.

Tisserand, R. *The Art of Aromatherapy*, C.W. Daniel, 1983.

Valnet, Dr J. *Aromatherapie*, Libraire Maloine, Paris, 1975, (distributed in Britain by C.W. Daniel).

Valnet, Dr. J. *The Practice of Aromatherapy*, C.W. Daniel, 1980.

Wright, C. *The Wright Diet*, Piatkus, 1986.

Useful Addresses

Oils Suppliers

The following suppliers stock a range of high quality aromatherapy grade oils. However, Kittywake, Bodytreats and Norman & Germaine Rich stock a selection of separately labelled organically produced oils – from plants grown without the use of chemical fertilizers and poisonous sprays.

Kittywake Oils,
Cae Kitty,
Taliaris,
Llandeilo,
Dyfed, SA19 7DP

Bodytreats Ltd.,
15 Approach Road,
Raynes Park,
London, SW20 8BA

Butterbur & Sage,
101 Highgrove Street,
Reading, RG1 5EJ

Norman & Germaine Rich,
2 Coval Gardens,
London, SW14 7DG

The Tisserand Institute,
P.O. Box 746,
Hove,
East Sussex, BN3 3XA

Aromatherapy Training Courses
For a prospectus of Aromatherapy courses write to:

The Tisserand Institute,
P.O. Box 746,
Hove,
East Sussex, BN3 3XA

Massage Courses
Clare Maxwell-Hudson,
87 Dartmouth Road,
London, NW2 4BR

For a prospectus of in-depth remedial massage courses, write to:

The Northern Institute of Massage,
100 Waterloo Road,
Blackpool,
Lancs, FY4 1AW

Aromatherapy Associations
For a list of qualified practising aromatherpists in your area, send a stamped addressed envelope to:

International Federation of Aromatherapists,
4 East Mearn Road,
Dulwich,
London

International Federation of Aromatherapists,
c/o Allison Russell,
35 Bydown Street,
Neutral Bay,
New South Wales 2089,
Australia

American Aromatherapy Association,
P. O. Box 3609,
Culver City,
California 90231,
U.S.A.

The Pegasus Foundation

If you are interested in spiritual healing, meditation and other esoteric subjects, contact the following organisation. They will be pleased to send details of their courses and seminars.

The Pegasus Foundation,
Runnings Park,
Croft Bank,
West Malvern,
Worcestershire,
WR14 4BP

Hyperactive Children's Support Group

If you would like to contact the Hyperactive Children's Support Group as mentioned in Chapter 3, send a stamped addressed envelope to:

HACSG,
71 Whyke Lane,
Chichester,
West Sussex, PO22 OBH

Music tapes

Relaxing music tapes are available from:

New World Cassettes,
FREEPOST,
Strawberry Vale,
Twickenham, TW1 1BR

Bach Flower Remedies

If you have difficulty obtaining authentic Bach Flower Remedies as discovered by Dr Edward Bach, send a stamped addressed envelope for a price list and information leaflet to:

The Bach Centre,
Mount Vernon,
Sotwell,
Oxfordshire, OX10 OPZ

Index